**Copyright © 2020 by Marie Tinsley -All rights reserved.**

No part of this publication may be reproduced, distributed, or transmitted in any form or by any means, including photocopying, recording, or other electronic or mechanical methods, without the prior written permission of the publisher, except in the case of brief quotations embodied in reviews and certain other non-commercial uses permitted by copyright law.

This Book is provided with the sole purpose of providing relevant information on a specific topic for which every reasonable effort has been made to ensure that it is both accurate and reasonable. Nevertheless, by purchasing this Book you consent to the fact that the author, as well as the publisher, are in no way experts on the topics contained herein, regardless of any claims as such that may be made within. It is recommended that you always consult a professional prior to undertaking any of the advice or techniques discussed within.This is a legally binding declaration that is considered both valid and fair by both the Committee of Publishers Association and the American Bar Association and should be considered as legally binding within the United States.

# CONTENTS

# INTRODUCTION

There are no needs for special diets if you are diabetic. There whole myth about diabetics' patients needing some specially designed meal plan is bogus. While there is a need to eat healthily as a diabetic because eating unhealthy has many health risks, the same also applies to people who do not have diabetes. As a diabetic patient, eating healthy is not an option you can overlook; it is compulsory. Having a healthy eating balance requires several things, and one such thing is meal prep. Planning your meals days before is a vital step in ensuring that your meals are as healthy as they possibly can be. Meal preps and helping you save cooking time also help you plan and organize your meals, making it possible for you to eat the right type of food that contains the right nutrients. Eating healthy has so many health benefits – to those who suffer from diabetics and those who do not. While the nutritional needs of a diabetic is the same as that of a healthy person, there are some slight differences between the meals. Some of these differences include:

- Diabetics patients need to pay closer attention to the type of carbs they take.
- Diabetics patients need to reduce belly fat significantly.

In eating healthy as a person with diabetes, you need to understand that there is no need to eat bland food all in the name of eating healthy. You can have it all – the tasty meals that you love and the healthy diets. Meals meant for diabetics basically deal with planning meals ahead of time, eating the right proportion of food at the right time, and the right combination of nutrients. With meal prep, you can quickly achieve the best of both worlds: excellent and tasty food and save time. You see, many people often run away from cooking because of the time it takes to make meals. If you are the busy type with loads of work commitment, then you have so much work on your plate that the mere thought of cooking makes you sick. That is where meal prep comes into play. Meal prep means preparing whole meals or dishes ahead of schedule. The nutritional benefits of meal prep should never be lost on you or anyone for that matter. Aside from helping you save time, meal preps help you reduce portion sizes, help you eat healthier, and make better meal choices over the long term.

**There are various ways to meal prep, even as a person with diabetes. These meal-prep ways include:**
- **Batch cooking**: This involves making large batches of a particular recipe, then diving it into individual portions that you can freeze and eat over the next few days or few weeks. For example, you can prepare large portions of Mediterranean recipes and then split them into small portions that you can eat later.

- **Ready-to-cook ingredients**: This is one of the most time-effective meal-prep methods. All you do is prepare the ingredients needed to prepare specific meals ahead of time.

- **Make-ahead meals:** These are complete meals that you cook in advance. After cooking, all you need to do is refrigerate the meal and reheat when it's time to eat it. If you're the type that doesn't have time to prepare dinner, this meal-prep method comes in very handy.

- **Individually portioned meals**: With this method, you prepare the meals fresh and portion them into individual grab-and-go portions that you refrigerate and eat over the next few days or weeks. In planning, you need to be sure of the type of meal-prep method that works for you. If the batch cooking method is what will be best for you, then stick with that method. If it's the ready-to-cook ingredients method, use it. The goal is to save time while eating healthy. With meal prep and diabetic meals, you must have various meals that you prepare and use different cooking methods. Using the one cooking method and preparing just one type of meal, you are likely to get bored with the cooking and recipes you use. Before we delve into the different tantalizing recipes in this book, let us demystify some myths people have about meals for a diabetic.

**Diabetics diet: The myths**

➢ **Myth 1**: Sugar is bad for a person with diabetes all the time: I am sure you must have heard this so many times: never eat sugar! Don't get close to sugar! Anything that contains sugar should never get a whiff from you; talk more of a taste! That is not true. Agreed, the sugar intake must be reduced – as so should every other person. But that does not mean you have to avoid sugar completely. All you need is to plan appropriately and limit, as much as you can, hidden in your meals. You can still have some of your sweets; they have to be in a healthy diet plan.

➢ **Myth 2:** A high-protein diet is the best: Too much protein, especially animal protein, can lead to insulin resistance, researchers have discovered. And insulin resistance is what diabetic patients are fighting against. This doesn't mean the protein is harmful. What it means is that we should balance the amount of protein we take with carbs and healthy fats.

> **Myth 3:** Diabetic meals are bland: There is nothing farther from the truth than this. The erroneous belief that diabetic diets make people cringe when they hear words such as "eat healthy." Also, there are no 'special' diabetic meals. What people often call diabetic meals are healthy, everyday meals that everyone should be eating.

> **Myth 4:** Reduce your carbs intake drastically: Starchy carbs are bad for your health, that is a fact. But that doesn't mean there are no other forms of carbs that a diabetic patient can eat. There are carbs gotten from whole grains that you can have. Carbs from whole grains are rich in fiber and digests slowly. And due to the fiber-richness of these carbs (the whole grain carbs), the blood sugar level becomes even.

**Diabetics Diet: The Facts**
> Eat more healthy fats, those gotten from nuts, flax seeds, olive oil, avocadoes, and fish oils.
> Eat less packaged foods, fast foods, and food high in sugar; sweets and chips should be reduced.
> Eat more high-quality protein; more fish, eggs, unsweetened yogurts, and beans.
> Eat less refined pasta and rice and sugary cereals.
> Eat more high-fiber meals, pieces of bread made from whole grains.
> Eat less red meat and processed meats.
> Eat more fruits and vegetables, especially leafy vegetables.
> Eat fewer foods that replace fat with more sugar. Examples of such foods include those 'fat-free' yogurts that have replaced fat with more sugar.

When meal prepping, to enjoy the wholesome benefits, you must do the following:
• **Have a schedule and stick to it**: One of the hardest parts of cooking is shopping. Going to the grocery store or market can be time-exhausting. To make the best of your meal prepping, schedule time to go to the market to shop for all you need for the meal prep. You also need, in addition to the prepared schedule, stick to the plan you have created. The plan is your choice, so you should design it to fit into your weekly routine.

• **Have recipe combinations**: Like I said earlier, having just one set of recipes will bore you and make the planning and cooking process tiring. With the right combination of healthy recipes, you become more effective in planning and executing meal plans. The recipes would also have to involve a variety of cooking methods, some smoking recipes, some boiling recipes, some baking, some uncooked recipes as well. Having various cooking methods ensures that you have sumptuous meals to eat and have fun planning and cooking them. Also, different cooking methods offer different flavors and tastes.

- **Designate prep time and cook time**: Apart from going to the grocery store, you also need to make time to plan and cook. It would help if you started cooking with recipes that require long cook time before cooking other meals that don't need as much time.Also, it is crucial, when going grocery shopping, to have a detailed list of what you need and the departments they are sold. When you organize your list correctly, you avoid going back and forth in the grocery store, looking for one condiment or the other.

**What You Will Get From This Book**

There are a plethora of recipe books out there. So, you might be wondering what makes this book so different. Well, several contents stand this book out.

- **The recipes are easy to follow through on**: The joy of every cook, every chef who writes a cookbook is seeing the readers make good the recipes he/she had curated for them. And one of the best ways to create recipe books that the everyday man, woman, boy, and girl can follow through is making the words easy to understand and the pictures clear. There are very few culinary jargon in this, making it super-easy to understand and follow through. The pictures that proceed with each recipe and follow-through cooking instructions are crisp and clear. The pictures clearly show what the recipes look like – and to a large extent, give you an idea on how they might taste.

- **The recipes are categorized**: The recipes in this book are categorized based on mealtimes, cook time, and cooking methods. You need to know what you will be having for dinner, breakfast, and lunch with meal prep. Also, you need to know what dessert will be. I have done well to arrange these recipes based on all the different meal times so that it is easier for you, when planning and preparing for your meals, to know what to prepare when and how to go about cooking these meals. Also, the recipes are categorized based on cooking methods. You don't want to use one cooking method all through your meal prep; it can get very boring when you do. Therefore, there are healthy smoking recipes, healthy baking recipes, and the likes. You can easily shuffle the cooking methods while still eating healthy and having fun planning, shopping and cooking meals. The recipes are also categorized based on the cooking time. You wouldn't want to start cooking first a recipe that takes only three minutes to prepare and leave out those that take more than an hour to prepare for later.

- **These recipes give you room to experiment**: I am a firm believer that cooking is as artistic as painting, as creative as writing, and therefore should be fun. The diabetic recipes in this book, which range from the cottage cheese crab to the roasted cauliflower tacos are experimental as they are tasty. As I was experimental in curating these recipes in this same vein, I also want you to try out new recipes on your own. There are no hard and fast rules with cooking. You are either doing right, or you are doing it right. Take your time, have fun with these recipes – with the planning and the cooking. There is so much you can do with these recipes; all you have to do is be free and experiment. You will get some meals wrong. But that shouldn't stop you from trying your hands with these recipes. Take your time. Even when they don't come out as expected, keep at it. As you go through these recipes, allow your creative genius to come forth. Create magic.

# BREAKFAST RECIPES

## Spiced Overnight Oats

Servings: 6     Cooking Time: None
**Ingredients:**
- 2 cups old-fashioned oats
- 1 cup fat-free milk
- 1 tablespoon vanilla extract
- 1 teaspoon liquid stevia extract
- 1 teaspoon ground cinnamon
- ¼ teaspoon ground nutmeg
- ½ cup toasted walnuts, chopped

**Directions:**
Stir together the oats, milk, vanilla extract, liquid stevia extract, cinnamon, and nutmeg in a large bowl.     Cover and chill overnight until thick.     Stir in the yogurt just before serving and spoon into cups.     Top with chopped walnuts and fresh fruit to serve.
**Nutrition Info:**Calories 140, Total Fat 7.1g, Saturated Fat 0.5g, Total Carbs 12.7g, Net Carbs 10.4g, Protein 5.6g, Sugar 2.6g, Fiber 2.3g, Sodium 23mg

## Almond & Berry Smoothie

Servings: 1     Cooking Time: 0 Minute
**Ingredients:**
- ⅔ cup frozen raspberries
- ½ cup frozen banana, sliced
- ½ cup almond milk (unsweetened)
- 3 tablespoons almonds, sliced
- ¼ teaspoon ground cinnamon
- ⅛ teaspoon vanilla extract
- ¼ cup blueberries
- 1 tablespoon coconut flakes (unsweetened)

**Directions:**
Put the Ingredients in a blender except coconut flakes. Pulse until smooth.     Top with the coconut flakes before serving.
**Nutrition Info:**Calories 360 Total Fat 19 g Saturated Fat 3 g Cholesterol 0 mg Sodium 89 mg Total Carbohydrate 46 g Dietary Fiber 14 g Total Sugars 21 g Protein 9 g Potassium 736 mg

## Keto Low Carb Crepe

Servings: 2     Cooking Time: 4 Minutes
**Ingredients:**
- 2 eggs
- 1 egg white
- 1 tbsp unsalted butter
- 1 1/3 tbsp cream cheese
- 2/3 tbsp psyllium husk

**Directions:**
preparation the batter and for this, put all the ingredients in a bowl, except for butter, and then whisk by using a stick blender until smooth and very liquid.     Bring out a skillet pan, put it over medium heat, add ½ tbsp butter and when it melts, pour in half of the batter, spread evenly, and cook until the top has firmed.     Carefully flip the crepe, then continue cooking for 2 minutes until

cooked and then move it to a plate.     Add remaining butter and when it melts, cook another crepe in the same manner and then serve.
**Nutrition Info:**118 Cal 9.4 g Fats 6.5 g Protein 1 g Net Carb 0.9 g Fiber

## Cinnamon Oat Pancakes

Servings: 6     Cooking Time: 15 Minutes
**Ingredients:**
- 1 cup old-fashioned oats
- 1 cup whole-wheat flour
- 2 teaspoons baking powder
- 1 teaspoon salt
- 1 ½ cups fat-free milk
- ¼ cup canola oil
- 2 large eggs, whisked
- 1 teaspoon lemon juice
- ½ to 1 teaspoon liquid stevia extract

**Directions:**
Combine the oats, flour, baking powder, and salt in a medium mixing bowl.     In a separate bowl, stir together the milk, canola oil, eggs, lemon juice, and stevia extract. Stir the wet ingredients into the dry until just combined. Heat a large skillet or griddle to medium-high heat and grease with cooking spray.     Spoon the batter in ¼ cups into the skillet and cook until bubbles form on the surface. Flip the pancakes and cook to brown on the other side. Slide onto a plate and repeat with the remaining batter. Store the extra pancakes in an airtight container and reheat in the microwave or oven.
**Nutrition Info:**Calories 230, Total Fat 11.4g, Saturated Fat 1.3g, Total Carbs 24.3g, Net Carbs 23g, Protein 7.1g, Sugar 3.3g, Fiber 1.3g, Sodium 446mg

## Yogurt And Kale Smoothie

Servings: 1
**Ingredients:**
- 1 cup whole milk yogurt
- 1 cup baby kale greens
- 1 pack stevia
- 1 tablespoon MCT oil
- 1 tablespoon sunflower seeds
- 1 cup of water

**Directions:**
Add listed ingredients to the blender     Blend until you have a smooth and creamy texture     Serve chilled and enjoy!
**Nutrition Info:**Calories: 329; Fat: 26g; Carbohydrates: 15g; Protein: 11g

## Healthy Carrot Muffins

Servings: 8     Cooking Time: 40 Minutes
**Ingredients:**
- Dry ingredients
- Tapioca starch – ¼ cup
- Baking soda – 1 teaspoon
- Cinnamon – 1 tablespoon

- Cloves – ¼ teaspoon
- Wet ingredients
- Vanilla extract – 1 teaspoon
- Water – 11/2 cups
- Carrots (shredded) – 11/2 cups
- Almond flour – 1¾ cups
- Granulated sweetener of choice – 1/2 cup
- Baking powder – 1 teaspoon
- Nutmeg – 1 teaspoon
- Salt – 1 teaspoon
- Coconut oil – 1/3 cup
- Flax meal – 4 tablespoons
- Banana (mashed) – 1 medium

**Directions:**
Begin by heating the oven to 350F. Get a muffin tray and position paper cups in all the moulds. Arrange aside. Get a small glass bowl and put half a cup of water and flax meal. Allow this rest for about 5 minutes. Your flax egg is prepared. Get a large mixing bowl and put in the almond flour, tapioca starch, granulated sugar, baking soda, baking powder, cinnamon, nutmeg, cloves, and salt. Mix well to combine. Conform a well in the middle of the flour mixture and stream in the coconut oil, vanilla extract, and flax egg. Mix well to conform a mushy dough. Then put in the chopped carrots and mashed banana. Mix until well-combined. Make use of a spoon to scoop out an equal amount of mixture into 8 muffin cups. Position the muffin tray in the oven and allow it to bake for about 40 minutes. Extract the tray from the microwave and allow the muffins to stand for about 10 minutes. Extract the muffin cups from the tray and allow them to chill until they reach room degree of hotness and coldness. Serve and enjoy!
**Nutrition Info:**Calories: 189 calories per serving; Fat 13.9 g; Protein 3.8 g; Carbs 17.3 g

## Breakfast Smoothie Bowl With Fresh Berries

Servings: 2     Cooking Time: 5 Minutes
**Ingredients:**
- Almond milk (unsweetened) – 1/2 cup
- Psyllium husk powder – 1/2 teaspoon
- Strawberries (chopped) – 2 ounces
- Coconut oil – 1 tablespoon
- Crushed ice – 3 cups
- Liquid stevia – 5 to 10 drops
- Pea protein powder – 1/3 cup

**Directions:**
Begin by taking a blender and adding in the mashed ice cubes. Allow them to rest for about 30 seconds. Then put in the almond milk, shredded strawberries, pea protein powder, psyllium husk powder, coconut oil, and liquid stevia. Blend well until it turns into a smooth and creamy puree. Vacant the prepared smoothie into 2 glasses. Cover with coconut flakes and pure and neat strawberries.
**Nutrition Info:**Calories: 166 calories per serving; Fat – 9.2 g; Carbs – 4.1 g; Protein – 17.6 g

## Keto Creamy Bacon Dish

Servings: 2     Cooking Time: 5 Minutes
**Ingredients:**

- ½ tsp dried basil
- ½ tsp minced garlic
- ½ tsp tomato paste
- 2 oz unsalted butter, softened
- 3 slices of bacon, chopped

**Directions:**
Bring out a skillet pan, put it over medium heat, add 1 tbsp butter and when it starts to melts, add chopped bacon and cook for 5 minutes. Then remove the pan from heat, add remaining butter, along with basil and tomato paste, season with salt and black pepper and stir until well mixed. Move bacon butter into an airtight container, cover with the lid, and refrigerate for 1 hour until solid.
**Nutrition Info:**150 Cal 16 g Fats 1 g Protein 0.5 g Net Carb 1 g Fiber

## Egg "dough" In A Pan

Servings: 2     Cooking Time: 4 Minutes
**Ingredients:**
- ¼ tsp salt
- ½ of medium red bell pepper, chopped
- 1/8 tsp ground black pepper
- 2 eggs
- 2 tbsp chopped chives

**Directions:**
Turn on the oven, then set it to 350 degrees F and let it preheat. In the meantime, crack eggs in a bowl, add remaining ingredients and whisk until combined. Bring out a small heatproof dish, pour in egg mixture, and bake for 5 to 8 minutes until set. When done, cut it into two squares and then serve.
**Nutrition Info:**87 Cal 5.4 g Fats 7.2 g Protein 1.7 g Net Carb 0.7 g Fiber

## Greek Chicken Breast

Servings: 4     Cooking Time: 25 Minutes
**Ingredients:**
- 4 chicken breast halves, skinless and boneless
- 1 cup extra virgin olive oil
- 1 lemon, juiced
- 2 teaspoons garlic, crushed
- 1 and 1/2 teaspoons black pepper
- 1/3 teaspoon paprika

**Directions:**
Cut 3 slits in the chicken breast     Take a small bowl and whisk in olive oil, salt, lemon juice, garlic, paprika, pepper and whisk for 30 seconds     Place chicken in a large bowl and pour marinade     Rub the marinade all over using your hand     Refrigerate overnight     Preheat grill to medium heat and oil the grate     Cook chicken in the grill until center is no longer pink     Serve and enjoy!
**Nutrition Info:**Calories: 644; Fat: 57g; Carbohydrates: 2g; Protein: 27g

## Eggs Florentine

Servings: 2     Cooking Time: 10 Minutes
**Ingredients:**
- 1 cup washed, fresh spinach leaves

- 2 tbsp freshly grated parmesan cheese
- Sea salt and pepper
- 1 tbsp white vinegar
- 2 eggs

**Directions:**

Cook the spinach the microwave or steam until wilted. Sprinkle with parmesan cheese and seasoning. Slice into bite-size pieces    Simmer a pan of water and add the vinegar. Stir quickly with a spoon.    Break an egg into the center. Turn off the heat and cover until set. Repeat with the second egg.    Place the eggs on top of the spinach and serve.

**Nutrition Info:**180 cal.10g fat 7g protein 5g carbs.

## Healthy Baked Eggs

Servings: 6    Cooking Time: 1 Hour

**Ingredients:**
- Olive oil – 1 tablespoon
- Garlic – 2 cloves
- Eggs – 8 large
- Sea salt – 1/2 teaspoon
- Shredded mozzarella cheese (medium-fat) – 3 cups
- Olive oil spray
- Onion (chopped) – 1 medium
- Spinach leaves – 8 ounces
- Half-and-half – 1 cup
- Black pepper – 1 teaspoon
- Feta cheese – 1/2 cup

**Directions:**

Begin by heating the oven to 375F.    Get a glass baking dish and grease it with olive oil spray. Arrange aside. Now take a nonstick pan and pour in the olive oil. Position the pan on allows heat and allows it heat. Immediately you are done, toss in the garlic, spinach, and onion. Prepare for about 5 minutes. Arrange aside. You can now Get a large mixing bowl and add in the half, eggs, pepper, and salt. Whisk thoroughly to combine. Put in the feta cheese and chopped mozzarella cheese (reserve 1/2 cup of mozzarella cheese for later).    Put the egg mixture and prepared spinach to the prepared glass baking dish. Blend well to combine. Drizzle the reserved cheese over the top.    Bake the egg mix for about 45 minutes.    Extract the baking dish from the oven and allow it to stand for 10 minutes.    Dice and serve!

**Nutrition Info:**Calories: 323 calories per serving; Fat 22.3 g; Protein  22.6 g; Carbs 7.9 g

## Quick Low-carb Oatmeal

Servings: 2    Cooking Time: 15 Minutes

**Ingredients:**
- Almond flour – 1/2 cup
- Flax meal – 2 tablespoons
- Cinnamon (ground) – 1 teaspoon
- Almond milk (unsweetened) – 11/2 cups
- Salt – as per taste
- Chia seeds – 2 tablespoons
- Liquid stevia – 10 – 15 drops
- Vanilla extract – 1 teaspoon

**Directions:**

Begin by taking a large mixing bowl and adding in the coconut flour, almond flour, ground cinnamon, flax seed powder, and chia seeds. Mix properly to combine. Position a stockpot on a low heat and add in the dry ingredients. Also add in the liquid stevia, vanilla extract, and almond milk. Mix well to combine.    Prepare the flour and almond milk for about 4 minutes. Add salt if needed.    Move the oatmeal to a serving bowl and top with nuts, seeds, and pure and neat berries.

**Nutrition Info:**Calories: calories per serving; Protein – 11.7 g; Fat – 24.3 g; Carbs – 16.7 g

## Balsamic Chicken

Servings: 6    Cooking Time: 25 Minutes

**Ingredients:**
- 6 chicken breast halves, skinless and boneless
- 1 teaspoon garlic salt
- Ground black pepper
- 2 tablespoons olive oil
- 1 onion, thinly sliced
- 14 and 1/2 ounces tomatoes, diced
- 1/2 cup balsamic vinegar
- 1 teaspoon dried basil
- 1 teaspoon dried oregano
- 1 teaspoon dried rosemary
- 1/2 teaspoon dried thyme

**Directions:**

Season both sides of your chicken breasts thoroughly with pepper and garlic salt    Take a skillet and place it over medium heat    Add some oil and cook your seasoned chicken for 3-4 minutes per side until the breasts are nicely browned    Add some onion and cook for another 3-4 minutes until the onions are browned    Pour the diced up tomatoes and balsamic vinegar over your chicken and season with some rosemary, basil, thyme, and rosemary    Simmer the chicken for about 15 minutes until they are no longer pink    Take an instant-read thermometer and check if the internal temperature gives a reading of 165 degrees Fahrenheit If yes, then you are good to go!

**Nutrition Info:**Calories: 196; Fat: 7g; Carbohydrates: 7g; Protein: 23g

## Vegetable Noodles Stir-fry

Servings: 4    Cooking Time: 40 Minutes

**Ingredients:**
- White sweet potato – 1 pound
- Zucchini – 8 ounces
- Garlic cloves (finely chopped) – 2 large
- Vegetable broth – 2 tablespoons
- Salt – as per taste
- Carrots – 8 ounces
- Shallot (finely chopped) – 1
- Red chili (finely chopped) – 1
- Olive oil – 1 tablespoon
- Pepper – as per taste

**Directions:**

Begin by scrapping the carrots and sweet potato.    Make Use a spiralizer to make noodles out of the sweet potato and carrots.    Rinse the zucchini thoroughly and spiralize it as well.    Get a large skillet and position it on

a high flame. Stream in the vegetable broth and allow it to come to a boil. Toss in the spiralized sweet potato and carrots. Then put in the chili, garlic, and shallots. Stir everything using tongs and cook for some minutes. Transfer the vegetable noodles into a serving platter and generously spice with pepper and salt. Finalize by sprinkling olive oil over the noodles. Serve while hot!
**Nutrition Info:**Calories: 169 calories per serving; Fat 3.7 g; Protein 3.6 g; Carbs – 31.2 g

## Cucumber & Yogurt

Servings: 1    Cooking Time: 0 Minute
**Ingredients:**
- 1 cup low-fat yogurt
- ½ cup cucumber, diced
- ¼ teaspoon lemon zest
- ¼ teaspoon lemon juice
- ¼ teaspoon fresh mint, chopped
- Salt to taste

**Directions:**
Mix all the Ingredients in a jar.    Refrigerate and serve.
**Nutrition Info:**Calories 164 Total Fat 4 g Saturated Fat 2 g Cholesterol 15 mg Sodium 318 mg Total Carbohydrate 19 g Dietary Fiber 1 g Total Sugars 18 g Protein 13 g Potassium 683 mg

## Eggs Baked In Peppers

Servings: 4    Cooking Time: 25 Minutes
**Ingredients:**
- 4 medium bell peppers, assorted
- 1 cup shredded low-fat cheddar cheese
- 8 large eggs
- Salt and pepper
- Fresh chopped parsley, to serve

**Directions:**
Preheat the oven to 400°F and slice the peppers in half. Remove the seeds and pith from each pepper and place them cut-side up in a baking dish large enough to fit them all.    Divide the shredded cheese among the pepper halves and crack an egg into each.    Season with salt and pepper then bake for 20 to 25 minutes until done to your liking.    Garnish with fresh chopped parsley to serve.
**Nutrition Info:**Calories 260, Total Fat 16.3g, Saturated Fat 6.6g, Total Carbs 10.9g, Net Carbs 9.3g, Protein 20.8g, Sugar 6.8g, Fiber 1.6g, Sodium 374mg

## Easy Egg Scramble

Servings: 1    Cooking Time: 10 Minutes
**Ingredients:**
- 2 large eggs
- 1 tablespoon fat-free milk
- Salt and pepper
- ¼ cup diced green pepper
- 2 tablespoons diced onion
- ¼ cup diced tomatoes

**Directions:**
Whisk together the eggs, milk, salt, and pepper in a small bowl.    Heat a medium skillet over medium-high heat and grease with cooking spray.    Add the green pepper

and onion then cook for 2 to 3 minutes.    Spoon the veggies into a bowl then reheat the skillet.    Pour in the egg mixture and cook until the eggs start to thicken. Spoon in the cooked veggies and diced tomatoes.    Stir the mixture and cook until the egg is set and scrambled. Serve hot.
**Nutrition Info:**Calories 170, Total Fat 10.1g, Saturated Fat 3.1g, Total Carbs 6.3g, Net Carbs 4.9g, Protein 13.9g, Sugar 4.1g, Fiber 1.4g, Sodium 152mg

## Bacon And Chicken Garlic Wrap

Servings: 4    Cooking Time: 10 Minutes
**Ingredients:**
- 1 chicken fillet, cut into small cubes
- 8-9 thin slices bacon, cut to fit cubes
- 6 garlic cloves, minced

**Directions:**
Preheat your oven to 400 degrees F    Line a baking tray with aluminum foil    Add minced garlic to a bowl and rub each chicken piece with it    Wrap bacon piece around each garlic chicken bite    Secure with toothpick Transfer bites to the baking sheet, keeping a little bit of space between them    Bake for about 15-20 minutes until crispy    Serve and enjoy!
**Nutrition Info:**Calories: 260; Fat: 19g; Carbohydrates: 5g; Protein: 22g

## Strawberry Puff Pancake

Servings: 4    Cooking Time: 20 Minutes
**Ingredients:**
- 3 eggs, large
- 1/8 teaspoon cinnamon, ground
- 1 cup strawberry, sliced
- 3/4 cup milk, fat-free
- What you will need from the store cupboard:
- 1 teaspoon vanilla extract
- ¾ cup of all-purpose flour
- 2 tablespoons of butter
- 1 tablespoon cornstarch
- ½ cup of water
- 1/8 teaspoon salt

**Directions:**
Keep the butter in a pie plate and keep in an oven for 4 to 5 minutes.    In the meantime, whisk the vanilla, milk, and eggs in a bowl.    Take another bowl and bring together the cinnamon, salt, and flour in it.    Whisk this into the egg mix until it blends well. Pour this into the plate.    Bake for 15 minutes. The sides should be golden brown and crisp.    Add the cornstarch in your saucepan. Stir the water in until it turns smooth.    Now add the strawberries. Cook while stirring till it thickens.    Mash the strawberries coarsely and serve with the pancake.
**Nutrition Info:**Calories 277, Carbohydrates 38g, Fiber 2g, Cholesterol 175mg, Total Fat 10g, Protein 9g, Sodium 187mg

## Egg Porridge

Servings: 1    Cooking Time: 10 Minutes
**Ingredients:**
- 2 organic free-range eggs

- 1/3 cup organic heavy cream without food additives
- 2 packages of your preferred sweetener
- 2 tbsp grass-fed butter ground organic cinnamon to taste

**Directions:**
In a bowl add the eggs, cream and sweetener, and mix together. Melt the butter in a saucepan over a medium heat. Lower the heat once the butter is melted. Combine together with the egg and cream mixture. While Cooking, mix until it thickens and curdles. When you see the first signs of curdling, remove the saucepan immediately from the heat. Pour the porridge into a bowl. Sprinkle cinnamon on top and serve immediately.
**Nutrition Info:** 604 cal 45g fat 8g protein 2.8g carbs.

## Chipotle Lettuce Chicken

Servings: 6     Cooking Time: 25 Minutes
**Ingredients:**
- 1 pound chicken breast, cut into strips
- Splash of olive oil
- 1 red onion, finely sliced
- 14 ounces tomatoes
- 1 teaspoon chipotle, chopped
- 1/2 teaspoon cumin
- Pinch of sugar
- Lettuce as needed
- Fresh coriander leaves
- Jalapeno chilies, sliced
- Fresh tomato slices for garnish
- Lime wedges

**Directions:**
Take a non-stick frying pan and place it over medium heat     Add oil and heat it up     Add chicken and cook until brown     Keep the chicken on the side     Add tomatoes, sugar, chipotle, cumin to the same pan and simmer for 25 minutes until you have a nice sauce     Add chicken into the sauce and cook for 5 minutes     Transfer the mix to another place     Use lettuce wraps to take a portion of the mixture and serve with a squeeze of lemon     Enjoy!
**Nutrition Info:** Calories: 332; Fat: 15g; Carbohydrates: 13g; Protein: 34g

## Breakfast Parfait

Servings: 2     Cooking Time: 0 Minute
**Ingredients:**
- 4 oz. unsweetened applesauce
- 6 oz. non-fat and sugar-free vanilla yogurt
- ¼ teaspoon pumpkin pie spice
- ¼ teaspoon honey
- 1 cup low-fat granola

**Directions:**
Mix the Ingredients except the granola in a bowl. Layer the mixture with the granola in a cup. Refrigerate before serving.
**Nutrition Info:** Calories 287 Total Fat 3 g Saturated Fat 1 g Cholesterol 28 mg Sodium 186 mg Total Carbohydrate 57 g Dietary Fiber 4 g Total Sugars 2 g Protein 8 g Potassium 4

## Oatmeal Blueberry Pancakes

Servings: 4     Cooking Time: 40 Minutes
**Ingredients:**
- ½ cup rolled oats
- ½ cup unsweetened almond milk
- ¼ cup unsweetened applesauce
- ¼ cup unsweetened vegan protein powder
- ½ tablespoon flax meal
- 1 teaspoon baking powder
- ½ teaspoon vanilla extract
- ¼ teaspoon baking soda
- ¼ teaspoon ground cinnamon
- 1/8 teaspoon salt
- ½ cup fresh blueberries

**Directions:**
Place all ingredients (except for blueberries) in a food processor and pulse until smooth. Transfer the mixture into a bowl and set aside for 5 minutes. Gently, fold in blueberries. Place a lightly greased medium skillet over medium heat until heated. Place desired amount of the mixture and cook for about 3–5 minutes per side. Repeat with the remaining mixture. Serve warm.
**Nutrition Info:** Calories 105 Total Fat 1.8 g Saturated Fat 0.2 g Cholesterol 0 mg Sodium 204 mg Total Carbs 15.4 g Fiber 2.2 g Sugar 5.2 g Protein 8 g

## Bulgur Porridge

Servings: 2     Cooking Time: 15 Minutes
**Ingredients:**
- 2/3 cup unsweetened soy milk
- 1/3 cup bulgur, rinsed
- Pinch of salt
- 1 ripe banana, peeled and mashed
- 2 kiwis, peeled and sliced

**Directions:**
In a pan, add the soy milk, bulgur, and salt over medium-high heat and bring to a boil. Adjust the heat to low and simmer for about 10 minutes. Remove the pan of bulgur from heat and immediately, stir in the mashed banana. Serve warm with the topping of kiwi slices.
**Nutrition Info:** Calories 223 Total Fat 2.3 g Saturated Fat 0.3 g Cholesterol 0 mg Sodium 126 mg Total Carbs 47.5 g Fiber 8.6 g Sugar 17.4 g Protein 7.1 g

## Turkey-broccoli Brunch Casserole

Servings: 6     Cooking Time: 20 Minutes
**Ingredients:**
- 2-1/2 cups turkey breast, cubed and cooked
- 16 oz. broccoli, chopped and drained
- 1-1/2 cups of milk, fat-free
- 1 cup cheddar cheese, low-fat, shredded
- 10 oz. cream of chicken soup. low sodium and low fat
- What you will need from the store cupboard:
- 8 oz. egg substitute
- ¼ teaspoon of poultry seasoning
- ¼ cup of sour cream, low fat
- ½ teaspoon pepper
- 1/8 teaspoon salt

- 2 cups of seasoned stuffing cubes
- Cooking spray

**Directions:**
Bring together the egg substitute, soup, milk, pepper, sour cream, salt, and poultry seasoning in a big bowl. Now stir in the broccoli, turkey, ¾ cup of cheese and stuffing cubes. Transfer to a baking dish. Apply cooking spray. Bake for 10 minutes. Sprinkle the remaining cheese. Bake for another 5 minutes. Keep it aside for 5 minutes. Serve.

**Nutrition Info:** Calories 303, Carbohydrates 26g, Fiber 3g, Sugar 0.8g, Cholesterol 72mg, Total Fat 7g, Protein 33g

## Cheesy Low-carb Omelet

Servings: 5     Cooking Time: 5 Minutes
**Ingredients:**
- 2 whole eggs
- 1 tablespoon water
- 1 tablespoon butter
- 3 thin slices salami
- 5 fresh basil leaves
- 5 thin slices, fresh ripe tomatoes
- 2 ounces fresh mozzarella cheese
- Salt and pepper as needed

**Directions:**
Take a small bowl and whisk in eggs and water. Take a non-stick Sauté pan and place it over medium heat, add butter and let it melt. Pour egg mixture and cook for 30 seconds. Spread salami slices on half of egg mix and top with cheese, tomatoes, basil slices. Season with salt and pepper according to your taste. Cook for 2 minutes and fold the egg with the empty half. Cover and cook on LOW for 1 minute. Serve and enjoy!

**Nutrition Info:** Calories: 451; Fat: 36g; Carbohydrates: 3g; Protein:33g

## Apple & Cinnamon Pancake

Servings: 4     Cooking Time: 10 Minutes
**Ingredients:**
- ¼ teaspoon ground cinnamon
- 1 ¾ cups Better Baking Mix
- 1 tablespoon oil
- 1 cup water
- 2 egg whites
- ½ cup sugar-free applesauce
- Cooking spray
- 1 cup plain yogurt
- Sugar substitute

**Directions:**
Blend the cinnamon and the baking mix in a bowl. Create a hole in the middle and add the oil, water, egg and applesauce. Mix well. Spray your pan with oil. Place it on medium heat. Pour ¼ cup of the batter. Flip the pancake and cook until golden. Serve with yogurt and sugar substitute.

**Nutrition Info:** Calories 231 Total Fat 6 g Saturated Fat 1 g Cholesterol 54 mg Sodium 545 mg Total Carbohydrate 37 g Dietary Fiber 4 g Total Sugars 1 g Protein 8 g Potassium 750 mg

## Guacamole Turkey Burgers

Servings: 3     Cooking Time: 15 Minutes
**Ingredients:**
- 12 oz. turkey, ground
- 1-1/2 avocados
- 2 teaspoons of juice from a lime
- ½ teaspoon cumin
- 1 red chili, chopped
- What you will need from the store cupboard:
- ½ teaspoon garlic powder
- ½ teaspoon onion powder
- 3 teaspoons of olive oil
- ½ teaspoon salt

**Directions:**
Mix the turkey with the cumin, chili, salt, garlic powder, and onion powder in a medium-sized bowl. Create 3 patties. Pour 3 teaspoons olive oil in a skillet and heat over medium heat. Now cook your patties. Make sure that both sides are brown. Make the guacamole in the meantime. Mash together the garlic powder, juice from lime and avocados in a bowl. Add salt for seasoning. Serve the burgers with guacamole on the patties.

**Nutrition Info:** Calories 316, Carbohydrates 9g, Fiber 8g, Sugar 0g, Cholesterol 80mg, Total Fat 21g, Protein 24g

## Ham And Goat Cheese Omelet

Servings: 1     Cooking Time: 10 Minutes
**Ingredients:**
- 1 slice of ham, chopped
- 4 egg whites
- 2 teaspoons of water
- 2 tablespoons onion, chopped
- 1 tablespoon parsley, minced
- What you will need from the store cupboard:
- 2 tablespoons green pepper, chopped
- 1/8 teaspoon pepper
- 2 tablespoons goat cheese, crumbled
- Cooking spray

**Directions:**
Whisk together the water, pepper and egg whites in a bowl till everything blends well. Stir in the green pepper, ham, and onion. Now heat your skillet over medium heat after applying the cooking spray. Pour in the egg white mix towards the edge. As it sets, push the cooked parts to the center. Allow the uncooked portions to flow underneath. Sprinkle the goat cheese to one side when there is no liquid egg. Now fold your omelet into half. Sprinkle the parsley.

**Nutrition Info:** Calories 143, Carbohydrates 5g, Fiber 1g, Sugar 0.3g, Cholesterol 27mg, Total Fat 4g, Protein 21g

## Strawberry & Spinach Smoothie

Servings: 2     Cooking Time: 15 Minutes
**Ingredients:**
- 1½ cups fresh strawberries, hulled and sliced
- 2 cups fresh baby spinach
- ½ cup fat-free plain Greek yogurt

- 1 cup unsweetened almond milk
- ¼ cup ice cubes

**Directions:**

In a high-speed blender, add all the ingredients and pulse until smooth. Pour into serving glasses and serve immediately.

**Nutrition Info:** Calories 96 Total Fat 2.3 g Saturated Fat 0.2 g Cholesterol 1 mg Total Carbs 12.3 g Sugar 7.7 g Fiber 3.9 g Sodium 144 mg Potassium 428 mg Protein 8.1 g

## Tomato And Zucchini Sauté

Servings: 6    Cooking Time: 43 Minutes

**Ingredients:**
- Vegetable oil – 1 tablespoon
- Tomatoes (chopped) – 2
- Green bell pepper (chopped) – 1
- Black pepper (freshly ground) – as per taste
- Onion (sliced) – 1
- Zucchini (peeled) – 2 pounds and cut into 1-inch-thick slices
- Salt – as per taste
- Uncooked white rice – ¼ cup

**Directions:**

Begin by getting a nonstick pan and putting it over low heat. Stream in the oil and allow it to heat through. Put in the onions and sauté for about 3 minutes. Then pour in the zucchini and green peppers. Mix well and spice with black pepper and salt. Reduce the heat and cover the pan with a lid. Allow the veggies cook on low for 5 minutes. While you're done, put in the water and rice. Place the lid back on and cook on low for 20 minutes.

**Nutrition Info:** Calories: 94 calories per serving; Fat – 2.8 g; Protein – 3.2 g; Carbs – 16.1 g

## Banana Matcha Breakfast Smoothie

Servings: 1    Cooking Time: None

**Ingredients:**
- 1 cup fat-free milk
- 1 medium banana, sliced
- ¼ cup frozen chopped pineapple
- ½ cup ice cubes
- 1 tablespoon matcha powder
- ¼ teaspoon ground cinnamon
- Liquid stevia extract, to taste

**Directions:**

Combine the ingredients in a blender. Pulse the mixture several times to chop the ingredients. Blend for 30 to 60 seconds until smooth and well combined. Sweeten to taste with liquid stevia extract, if desired. Pour into a glass and serve immediately.

**Nutrition Info:** Calories 230, Total Fat 0.4g, Saturated Fat 0.1g, Total Carbs 44.9g, Net Carbs 38g, Protein 12.6g, Sugar 30.9g, Fiber 6.9g, Sodium 135mg

## Tofu And Vegetable Scramble

Servings: 2    Cooking Time: 15 Minutes

**Ingredients:**
- Firm tofu (drained) – 16 ounces
- Sea salt – ½ teaspoon

- Garlic powder – 1 teaspoon
- Fresh coriander – for garnishing
- Red onion – 1/2 medium
- Cumin powder – 1 teaspoon
- Lemon juice – for topping
- Green bell pepper – 1 medium
- Garlic powder – 1 teaspoon
- Fresh coriander – for garnishing
- Red onion – 1/2 medium
- Cumin powder – 1 teaspoon
- Lemon juice – for topping

**Directions:**

Begin by preparing the ingredients. For this, you are to extract the seeds of the tomato and green bell pepper. Shred the onion, bell pepper, and tomato into small cubes. Get a small mixing bowl and position the fairly hard tofu inside it. Make use of your hands to break the fairly hard tofu. Arrange aside. Get a nonstick pan and add in the onion, tomato, and bell pepper. Mix and cook for about 3 minutes. Put the somewhat hard crumbled tofu to the pan and combine well. Get a small bowl and put in the water, turmeric, garlic powder, cumin powder, and chili powder. Combine well and stream it over the tofu and vegetable mixture. Allow the tofu and vegetable crumble cook with seasoning for 5 minutes. Continuously stir so that the pan is not holding the ingredients. Drizzle the tofu scramble with chili flakes and salt. Combine well. Transfer the prepared scramble to a serving bowl and give it a proper spray of lemon juice. Finalize by garnishing with pure and neat coriander. Serve while hot!

**Nutrition Info:** Calories: 238 calories per serving; Carbohydrates – 16.6 g; Fat – 11 g

## Basil And Tomato Baked Eggs

Servings: 4    Cooking Time: 15 Minutes

**Ingredients:**
- 1 garlic clove, minced
- 1 cup canned tomatoes
- ¼ cup fresh basil leaves, roughly chopped
- 1/2 teaspoon chili powder
- 1 tablespoon olive oil
- 4 whole eggs
- Salt and pepper to taste

**Directions:**

Preheat your oven to 375 degrees F    Take a small baking dish and grease with olive oil    Add garlic, basil, tomatoes chili, olive oil into a dish and stir    Crackdown eggs into a dish, keeping space between the two    Sprinkle the whole dish with salt and pepper    Place in oven and cook for 12 minutes until eggs are set and tomatoes are bubbling    Serve with basil on top    Enjoy!

**Nutrition Info:** Calories: 235; Fat: 16g; Carbohydrates: 7g; Protein: 14g

## Cream Cheese Pancakes

Servings: 1    Cooking Time: 5 Minutes

**Ingredients:**
- 2 oz cream cheese
- 2 eggs

- ½ tsp cinnamon
- 1 tbsp keto coconut flour
- ½ to 1 packet of Stevia

**Directions:**
Skillet with butter the pan or coconut oil on medium-high. Make them as you would normal pancakes. Cook and flip one side to cook the other side! Top with some butter and/or sugar-free syrup.

**Nutrition Info:**340 cal.30g fat 7g protein 3g carbs

## Chia And Coconut Pudding

Servings: 2     Cooking Time: 5 Minutes

**Ingredients:**
- Light coconut milk – 7 ounces
- Liquid stevia – 3 to 4 drops
- Kiwi – 1
- Chia seeds – ¼ cup
- Clementine – 1
- Shredded coconut (unsweetened)

**Directions:**
Begin by getting a mixing bowl and putting in the light coconut milk. Set in the liquid stevia to sweeten the milk. Combine well. Put the chia seeds to the milk and whisk until well-combined. Arrange aside. Scrape the clementine and carefully extract the skin from the wedges. Leave aside. Also, scrape the kiwi and dice it into small pieces. Get a glass vessel and gather the pudding. For this, position the fruits at the bottom of the jar; then put a dollop of chia pudding. Then spray the fruits and then put another layer of chia pudding. Finalize by garnishing with the rest of the fruits and chopped coconut.

**Nutrition Info:**Calories: 201 calories per serving; Protein – 5.4 g; Fat – 10 g; Carbs – 22.8 g

## Buckwheat Grouts Breakfast Bowl

Servings: 4     Cooking Time: 10 To 12 Minutes

**Ingredients:**
- 3 cups skim milk
- 1 cup buckwheat grouts
- ¼ cup chia seeds
- 2 teaspoons vanilla extract
- 1/2 teaspoon ground cinnamon
- Pinch salt
- 1 cup water
- 1/2 cup unsalted pistachios
- 2 cups sliced fresh strawberries
- ¼ cup cacao nibs (optional)

**Directions:**
In a large bowl, stir together the milk, groats, chia seeds, vanilla, cinnamon, and salt. Cover and refrigerate overnight. The next morning, transfer the soaked mixture to a medium pot and add the water. Bring to a boil over medium-high heat, reduce the heat to maintain a simmer, and cook for 10 to 12 minutes, until the buckwheat is tender and thickened. Transfer to bowls and serve, topped with the pistachios, strawberries, and cacao nibs (if using).

**Nutrition Info:**Calories: 340; Total fat: 8g; Saturated fat: 1g; Protein: 15g; Carbs: 52g; Sugar: 14g; Fiber: 10g; Cholesterol: 4mg; Sodium: 140mg

## Mashed Cauliflower

Servings: 6     Cooking Time: 10 Minutes

**Ingredients:**
- 1 cauliflower head
- 1/8 cup plain yogurt, skim milk or butter
- 1 red chili, diced
- 1 tomato, sliced
- ½ chopped onion
- What you will need from the store cupboard:
- 1 garlic clove, optional
- Salt and pepper
- Paprika to taste

**Directions:**
Steam the cauliflower till it becomes tender. You can steam with a garlic clove as well. Now cut your cauliflower into small pieces. Keep in your blender with yogurt, butter or milk. Season with pepper and salt. Whip until it gets smooth. Pour the cauliflower into a small baking dish. Sprinkle the paprika. Bake in the oven till it becomes bubbly.

**Nutrition Info:**Calories 57, Carbohydrates 12g, Total Fat 0g, Protein 4g, Fiber 5g, Sodium 91mg, Sugars 5g

## Quinoa Porridge

Servings: 2     Cooking Time: 20 Minutes

**Ingredients:**
- 1 cup dry quinoa, rinsed
- 1½ cups unsweetened almond milk
- 1 teaspoon vanilla extract
- 1 teaspoon ground cinnamon
- 2 tablespoons maple syrup
- 4 tablespoons peanut butter
- ¼ cup fresh strawberries, hulled and chopped
- ¼ cup fresh blueberries

**Directions:**
In a small pan, place quinoa, almond milk, vanilla extract, and cinnamon over medium heat and bring to a boil. Now, adjust the heat to low and simmer, covered for about 15 minutes or until all the liquid is absorbed. Remove the pan of quinoa from heat and stir in maple syrup and peanut butter. Serve warm with the topping of berries.

**Nutrition Info:**Calories 608 Total Fat 24 g Saturated Fat 4.2 g Cholesterol 0 mg Sodium 289 mg Total Carbs 81 g Fiber 10 g Sugar 17.9 g Protein 21.1 g

## Vanilla Mixed Berry Smoothie

Servings: 1     Cooking Time: None

**Ingredients:**
- 1 cup fat-free milk
- ½ cup nonfat Greek yogurt, plain
- ½ cup frozen blueberries
- ¼ cup frozen strawberries
- 3 to 4 ice cubes
- 1 teaspoon fresh lemon juice
- Liquid stevia extract, to taste

**Directions:**
Combine the ingredients in a blender. Pulse the mixture several times to chop the ingredients. Blend for 30 to 60 seconds until smooth and well combined.

Sweeten to taste with liquid stevia extract, if desired. Pour into a glass and serve immediately.
**Nutrition Info:**Calories 220, Total Fat 0.3g, Saturated Fat 0g, Total Carbs 31.6g, Net Carbs 28.3g, Protein 21.6g, Sugar 27.3g, Fiber 3.3g, Sodium 204mg

## Veggie Frittata

Servings: 6    Cooking Time: 25 Minutes
**Ingredients:**
- 1 tablespoon olive oil
- 1 large sweet potato, cut and peeled into thin slices
- 1 yellow squash, sliced
- 1 zucchini, sliced
- ½ of red bell pepper, seeded and sliced
- ½ of yellow bell pepper, seeded and sliced
- 8 eggs
- Salt and ground black pepper, as required
- 2 tablespoons fresh cilantro, chopped finely

**Directions:**
Preheat the oven to broiler.    over medium-low heat, cook the sweet potato for about 6-7 minutes.    Add the yellow squash, zucchini and bell peppers and cook for about 3-4 minutes.    Meanwhile, in a bowl, add the eggs, salt and black pepper and beat until well combined. Pour egg mixture over vegetables mixture.    Transfer the skillet in the oven and broil for about 3-4 minutes or until top becomes golden brown.    With a sharp knife, cut the frittata in desired size slices and serve with the garnishing of cilantro.
**Nutrition Info:**Calories 143 Total Fat 8.4 g Saturated Fat 2.2 g Cholesterol 218 mg Total Carbs 9.3 g Sugar 4.2 g Fiber 1.1 g Sodium 98 mg Potassium 408 mg Protein 8.9 g

## Cinnamon Rolls

Servings: 10    Cooking Time: 20 Minutes
**Ingredients:**
- 1 instant yeast packet
- 1 egg, large
- ¾ cups of whole milk
- 2-3/4 cups of flour
- 1 tablespoon ground cinnamon
- What you will need from the store cupboard:
- 4 tablespoons of butter, melted and unsalted
- ¾ teaspoon salt
- 2 tablespoons of maple syrup

**Directions:**
First, prepare your dough. Warm the milk and whisk in the yeast.    Keep it aside so that the yeast becomes foamy.    Beat the remaining butter, egg, flour, and salt until everything combines well.    Include ¼ cup flour. Knead your dough for a minute.    Line your cooker with parchment paper.    Create the filling. Create small rectangles with your dough and apply butter on top. Add cinnamon. Sprinkle butter on top    Roll the dough up. Cut into small pieces. Cook covered.    Take out and then whisk in the milk and maple syrup for the icing. Drizzle some milk over your rolls.
**Nutrition Info:**Calories 240, Carbohydrates 41g, Cholesterol 33mg, Total Fat 7g, Protein 4g, Fiber 4g, Sodium 254mg

## Whole-grain Pancakes

Servings: 4 To 6    Cooking Time: 15 Minutes
**Ingredients:**
- 2 cups whole-wheat pastry flour
- 4 teaspoons baking powder
- 2 teaspoons ground cinnamon
- 1/2 teaspoon salt
- 2 cups skim milk, plus more as needed
- 2 large eggs
- 1 tablespoon honey
- Nonstick cooking spray
- Maple syrup, for serving
- Fresh fruit, for serving

**Directions:**
In a large bowl, stir together the flour, baking powder, cinnamon, and salt.    Add the milk, eggs, and honey, and stir well to combine. If needed, add more milk, 1 tablespoon at a time, until there are no dry spots and you has a pourable batter.    Heat a large skillet over medium-high heat, and spray it with cooking spray. Using a ¼-cup measuring cup, scoop 2 or 3 pancakes into the skillet at a time. Cook for a couple of minutes, until bubbles form on the surface of the pancakes, flip, and cook for 1 to 2 minutes more, until golden brown and cooked through. Repeat with the remaining batter. Serve topped with maple syrup or fresh fruit.
**Nutrition Info:**Calories: 392; Total fat: 4g; Saturated fat: 1g; Protein: 15g; Carbs: 71g; Sugar: 11g; Fiber: 9g; Cholesterol: 95mg; Sodium: 396mg

## Granola With Fruits

Servings: 6    Cooking Time: 35 Minutes
**Ingredients:**
- 3 cups quick cooking oats
- 1 cup almonds, sliced
- ½ cup wheat germ
- 3 tablespoons butter
- 1 teaspoon ground cinnamon
- 1 cup honey
- 3 cups whole grain cereal flakes
- ½ cup raisins
- ½ cup dried cranberries
- ½ cup dates, pitted and chopped

**Directions:**
Preheat your oven to 325 degrees F.    Place the almonds on a baking sheet.    Bake for 15 minutes. Mix the wheat germ, butter, cinnamon and honey in a bowl.    Add the toasted almonds and oats.    Mix well. Spread on the baking sheet.    Bake for 20 minutes. Mix with the rest of the ingredients.    Let cool and serve.
**Nutrition Info:**Calories 210 Total Fat 7 g Saturated Fat 2 g Cholesterol 5 mg Sodium 58 mg Total Carbohydrate 36 g Dietary Fiber 4 g Total Sugars 2 g Protein 5 g Potassium 250 mg

## Egg Muffins

Servings: 6    Cooking Time: 20 Minutes
**Ingredients:**
- 1 tbsp green pesto
- 3 oz/75g shredded cheese

- 5 oz/150g cooked bacon
- 1 scallion, chopped
- 6 eggs

**Directions:**
You should set your oven to 350°F/175°C.    Place liners in a regular cupcake tin. This will help with easy removal and storage.    Beat the eggs with pepper, salt, and the pesto. Mix in the cheese.    Pour the eggs into the cupcake tin and top with the bacon and scallion.    Cook for 15-20 minutes

**Nutrition Info:**190 cal.15g fat 7g protein 4g carbs.

## Eggs On The Go

Servings: 4     Cooking Time: 5 Minutes

**Ingredients:**
- 4 oz/110g bacon, cooked
- Pepper
- Salt
- 12 eggs

**Directions:**
You should set your oven to 200°C.    Place liners in a regular cupcake tin. This will help with easy removal and storage.    Crack an egg into each of the cups and sprinkle some bacon onto each of them. Season with some pepper and salt.    Bake for 15 minutes, or until the eggs are set.

**Nutrition Info:**75 cal. 6g fat 8g protein 1g carbs.

## Breakfast Mix

Servings: 1     Cooking Time: 5 Minutes

**Ingredients:**
- 5 tbsp coconut flakes, unsweetened
- 7 tbsp hemp seeds
- 5 tbsp flaxseed, ground
- 2 tbsp sesame, ground
- 2 tbsp cocoa, dark, unsweetened

**Directions:**
Grind the sesame and flaxseed.    only grind the sesame seeds for a small period..    Mix all ingredients in a jar and shake it well.    Keep refrigerated until ready to eat. Serve softened with black coffee or even with still water and add coconut oil if you want to increase the fat content. It also blends well with cream or with mascarpone cheese.

**Nutrition Info:**150 cal.9g fat 8g protein 4g carbs.

## Lovely Porridge

Servings: 2     Cooking Time: Nil

**Ingredients:**
- 2 tablespoons coconut flour
- 2 tablespoons vanilla protein powder
- 3 tablespoons Golden Flaxseed meal
- 1 and 1/2 cups almond milk, unsweetened
- Powdered erythritol

**Directions:**
Take a bowl and mix in flaxseed meal, protein powder, coconut flour and mix well    Add mix to the saucepan (placed over medium heat)    Add almond milk and stir, let the mixture thicken    Add your desired amount of sweetener and serve    Enjoy!

**Nutrition Info:**Calories: 259; Fat: 13g; Carbohydrates: 5g; Protein: 16g

## Vegetable Omelet

Servings: 4     Cooking Time: 25 Minutes

**Ingredients:**
- 1/2 cup yellow summer squash, chopped
- 1/2 cup canned diced tomatoes with herbs, drained
- 1/2 ripe avocado, pitted and chopped
- 1/2 cup cucumber, chopped
- 2 eggs
- 2 tablespoons water
- Salt and pepper to taste
- 1 teaspoon dried basil, crushed
- Cooking spray
- 1/4 cup low-fat Monterey Jack cheese, shredded
- Chives, chopped

**Directions:**
In a bowl, mix the squash, tomatoes, avocado and cucumber.    In another bowl, mix the eggs, water, salt, pepper and basil.    Spray oil on a pan over medium heat.    Pour egg mixture on the pan.    Put the vegetable mixture on top of the egg.    Lift and fold. Cook until the egg has set.    Sprinkle cheese and chives on top.

**Nutrition Info:**Calories 128 Total Fat 6 g Saturated Fat 2 g Cholesterol 97 mg Sodium 357 mg Total Carbohydrate 7 g Dietary Fiber 3 g Total Sugars 4 g Protein 12 g Potassium 341 mg

## Vegetable Frittata

Servings: 2     Cooking Time: 20 Minutes

**Ingredients:**
- 1 cup mushrooms, sliced
- 4 eggs, beaten lightly
- 2 tablespoons onion, chopped
- 1/2 cup broccoli, chopped
- 1/4 cup cheddar cheese, shredded, low-fat
- What you will need from the store cupboard:
- 2 tablespoons green pepper, chopped
- Dash of pepper
- 1/8 teaspoon of salt
- Cooking spray

**Directions:**
Bring together all the ingredients in your bowl.    Coat your baking dish with cooking spray and pour everything into it.    Bake for 20 minutes and serve immediately.

**Nutrition Info:**Calories 230, Carbohydrates 6g, Fiber 1g, Sugar 0.2g, Cholesterol 386mg, Total Fat 14g, Protein 20g

## Egg-veggie Scramble

Servings: 2     Cooking Time: 3 Minutes

**Ingredients:**
- 1/4 tsp salt
- 1 tbsp unsalted butter
- 1/8 tsp ground black pepper
- 3 eggs, beaten
- 4 oz spinach

**Directions:**

Bring out a frying pan, put it over medium heat, add butter and when it melts, add spinach and cook for 5 minutes until leaves have wilted.    Then pour in eggs, season with salt and black pepper, and cook for 3 minutes until eggs have scramble to the desired level.
**Nutrition Info:**90 Cal 7 g Fats 5.6 g Protein; 0.7 g Net Carb 0.6 g Fiber

## Apple Omelet

Servings: 3      Cooking Time: 10 Minutes
**Ingredients:**
- 4 teaspoons olive oil, divided
- 2 small green apples, cored and sliced thinly
- ¼ teaspoon ground cinnamon
- Pinch of ground cloves
- Pinch of ground nutmeg
- 4 large eggs
- ¼ teaspoon organic vanilla extract
- Pinch of salt

**Directions:**
over medium-low heat in frying pan, heat 1 teaspoon Place the apple slices and sprinkle with spices.    Cook for about 4-5 minutes, flipping once halfway through. Meanwhile, in a bowl, add the eggs, vanilla extract and salt and beat until fluffy.     Add the remaining oil in the pan and let it heat completely.     Place the egg mixture over apple slices evenly and cook for about 3-5 minutes or until desired doneness.     Carefully, turn the pan over a serving plate and immediately, fold the omelet. Serve immediately.
**Nutrition Info:**Calories 228 Total Fat 13.2 g Saturated Fat 3 g Cholesterol 248 mg Total Carbs 21.3 g Sugar 16.1 g Fiber 3.8 g Sodium 145 mg Potassium 251 mg Protein 8.8 g

## Mix Veggie Fritters

Servings: 2      Cooking Time: 3 Minutes
**Ingredients:**
- ½ tsp nutritional yeast
- 1 oz chopped broccoli
- 1 zucchini, grated, squeezed
- 2 eggs
- 2 tbsp almond flour

**Directions:**
Wrap grated zucchini in a cheesecloth, twist it well to remove excess moisture, and then Put zucchini in a bowl. Add remaining ingredients, except for oil, and then whisk well until combined.     Bring out a skillet pan, put it over medium heat, add oil and when hot, drop zucchini mixture in four portions, shape them into flat patties and cook for 4 minutes per side until thoroughly cooked.
**Nutrition Info:**191 Cal 16.6 g Fats 9.6 g Protein 0.8 g Net Carb 0.2 g Fiber

## Millet Porridge

Servings: 4      Cooking Time: 25 Minutes
**Ingredients:**
- 1 cup millet, rinsed and drained
- Pinch of salt
- 3 cups water

- 2 tablespoons almonds, chopped finely
- 6-8 drops liquid stevia
- 1 cup unsweetened almond milk
- 2 tablespoons fresh blueberries

**Directions:**
In a nonstick pan, add the millet over medium-low heat and cook for about 3 minutes, stirring continuously. Add the salt and water and stir to combine    Increase the heat to medium and bring to a boil.     Cook for about 15 minutes.     Stir in the almonds, stevia and almond milk and cook for 5 minutes.     Top with the blueberries and serve.
**Nutrition Info:**Calories 219 Total Fat 4.5 g Saturated Fat 0.6 g Cholesterol 0 mg Total Carbs 38.2 g Sugar 0.6 g Fiber 5 g Sodium 92 mg Potassium 1721 mg Protein 6.4 g

## Steel-cut Oatmeal Bowl With Fruit And Nuts

Servings: 4      Cooking Time: 20 Minutes
**Ingredients:**
- 1 cup steel-cut oats
- 2 cups almond milk
- ¾ cup water
- 1 teaspoon ground cinnamon
- ¼ teaspoon salt
- 2 cups chopped fresh fruit, such as blueberries, strawberries, raspberries, or peaches
- 1/2 cup chopped walnuts
- ¼ cup chia seeds

**Directions:**
In a medium saucepan over medium-high heat, combine the oats, almond milk, water, cinnamon, and salt. Bring to a boil, reduce the heat to low, and simmer for 15 to 20 minutes, until the oats are softened and thickened. Top each bowl with 1/2 cup of fresh fruit, 2 tablespoons of walnuts, and 1 tablespoon of chia seeds before serving.
**Nutrition Info:**Calories: 288; Total fat: 11g; Saturated fat: 1g; Protein: 10g; Carbs: 38g; Sugar: 7g; Fiber: 10g; Cholesterol: 0mg; Sodium: 329mg

## Salty Macadamia Chocolate Smoothie

Servings: 1      Cooking Time: Nil
**Ingredients:**
- 2 tablespoons macadamia nuts, salted
- 1/3 cup chocolate whey protein powder, low  carb
- 1 cup almond milk, unsweetened

**Directions:**
Add the listed ingredients to your blender and blend until you have a smooth mixture    Chill and enjoy it!
**Nutrition Info:**Calories: 165; Fat: 2g; Carbohydrates: 1g; Protein: 12g

## Tofu & Zucchini Muffins

Servings: 6      Cooking Time: 40 Minutes
**Ingredients:**
- 12 ounces extra-firm silken tofu, drained and pressed
- ¾ cup unsweetened soy milk
- 2 tablespoons canola oil
- 1 tablespoon apple cider vinegar

- 1 cup whole-wheat pastry flour
- ½ cup chickpea flour
- 1 teaspoon baking powder
- ½ teaspoon baking soda
- 1 teaspoon smoked paprika
- 1 teaspoon onion powder
- 1 teaspoon salt
- ½ cup zucchini, chopped
- ¼ cup fresh chives, minced

**Directions:**
Preheat your oven to 400°F.    Line a 12-cup muffin tin with paper liners.    In a bowl, place tofu and with a fork, mash until smooth.    In the bowl of tofu, add almond milk, oil, and vinegar, and mix until slightly smooth. In a separate large bowl, add flours, baking powder, baking soda, spices, and salt, and mix well.    Transfer the mixture into muffin cups evenly.    Bake for approximately 35–40 minutes or until a toothpick inserted in the center comes out clean.    Remove the muffin tin from oven and place onto a wire rack to cool for about 10 minutes.    Carefully invert the muffins onto a platter and serve warm.

**Nutrition Info:**Calories 237 Total Fat 9 g Saturated Fat 1 g Cholesterol 0 mg Sodium 520 mg Total Carbs 2293.3 g Fiber 5.9 g Sugar 3.7 g Protein 11.1 g

## Savory Keto Pancake

Servings: 2    Cooking Time: 2 Minutes
**Ingredients:**
- ¼ cup almond flour
- 1 ½ tbsp unsalted butter
- 2 eggs
- 2 oz cream cheese, softened

**Directions:**
Bring out a bowl, crack eggs in it, whisk well until fluffy, and then whisk in flour and cream cheese until well combined.    Bring out a skillet pan, put it over medium heat, add butter and when it melts, drop pancake batter in four sections, spread it evenly, and cook for 2 minutes per side until brown.

**Nutrition Info:**166.8 Cal 15 g Fats 5.8 g Protein 1.8 g Net Car 0.8 g Fiber

## Sweet Potato Waffles

Servings: 2    Cooking Time: 20 Minutes
**Ingredients:**
- 1 medium sweet potato, peeled, grated and squeezed
- 1 teaspoon fresh thyme, minced
- 1 teaspoon fresh rosemary, minced
- 1/8 teaspoon red pepper flakes, crushed
- Salt and ground black pepper, as required

**Directions:**
Preheat the waffle iron and then grease it.    In a large bowl, add all ingredients and mix till well combined. Place half of the sweet potato mixture into preheated waffle iron and cook for about 8-10 minutes or until golden brown.    Repeat with the remaining mixture. Serve warm.

**Nutrition Info:**Calories 72 Total Fat 0.3 g Saturated Fat 0.1 g Cholesterol 0 mg Total Carbs 16.3 g Sugar 4.9 g

Fiber 3 g Sodium 28 mg Potassium 369 mg Protein 1.6 g

## Buckwheat Porridge

Servings: 2    Cooking Time: 15 Minutes
**Ingredients:**
- 1½ cups water
- 1 cup buckwheat groats, rinsed
- ¾ teaspoon vanilla extract
- ½ teaspoon ground cinnamon
- ¼ teaspoon salt
- 2 tablespoons maple syrup
- 1 ripe banana, peeled and mashed
- 1½ cups unsweetened soy milk
- 1 tablespoon peanut butter
- 1/3 cup fresh strawberries, hulled and chopped

**Directions:**
Place the water, buckwheat, vanilla extract, cinnamon, and salt in a pan and bring to a boil.    Now, adjust the heat to medium-low and simmer for about 6 minutes, stirring occasionally.    Stir in maple syrup, banana, and soy milk, and simmer, covered for about 6 minutes. Remove the pan of porridge from heat and stir in peanut butter.    Serve warm with the topping of strawberry pieces.

**Nutrition Info:**Calories 453 Total Fat 9.4 g Saturated Fat 1.7 g Cholesterol 0 mg Sodium 374 mg Total Carbs 82.8 g Fiber 9.4 g Sugar 28.8 g Protein 16.2 g

## Breakfast Sandwich

Servings: 2    Cooking Time: 0 Minutes
**Ingredients:**
- 2 oz/60g cheddar cheese
- 1/6 oz/30g smoked ham
- 2 tbsp butter
- 4 eggs

**Directions:**
Fry all the eggs and sprinkle the pepper and salt on them. Place an egg down as the sandwich base. Top with the ham and cheese and a drop or two of Tabasco.    Place the other egg on top and enjoy.

**Nutrition Info:**600 cal.50g fat 12g protein 7g carbs.

## Berry-oat Breakfast Bars

Servings: 12    Cooking Time: 25 Minutes
**Ingredients:**
- 2 cups fresh raspberries or blueberries
- 2 tablespoons sugar
- 2 tablespoons freshly squeezed lemon juice
- 1 tablespoon cornstarch
- 11/2 cups rolled oats
- 1/2 cup whole-wheat flour
- 1/2 cup walnuts
- ¼ cup chia seeds
- ¼ cup extra-virgin olive oil
- ¼ cup honey
- 1 large egg

**Directions:**
Preheat the oven to 350F.    In a small saucepan over medium heat, stir together the berries, sugar, lemon

juice, and cornstarch. Bring to a simmer. Reduce the heat and simmer for 2 to 3 minutes, until the mixture thickens. In a food processor or high-speed blender, combine the oats, flour, walnuts, and chia seeds. Process until powdered. Add the olive oil, honey, and egg. Pulse a few more times, until well combined. Press half of the mixture into a 9-inch square baking dish.    Spread the berry filling over the oat mixture. Add the remaining oat mixture on top of the berries. Bake for 25 minutes, until browned.    Let cool completely, cut into 12 pieces, and serve. Store in a covered container for up to 5 days.

**Nutrition Info:**Calories: 201; Total fat: 10g; Saturated fat: 1g; Protein: 5g; Carbs: 26g; Sugar: 9g; Fiber: 5g; Cholesterol: 16mg; Sodium: 8mg 30 MINUTES OR LESS • NUT FREE • VEGETARIAN

## Eggplant Omelet

Servings: 2    Cooking Time: 5 Minutes
**Ingredients:**
- 1 large eggplant
- 1 tbsp coconut oil, melted
- 1 tsp unsalted butter
- 2 eggs
- 2 tbsp chopped green onions

**Directions:**
Set the grill and let it preheat at the high setting.    In the meantime, Prepare the eggplant, and for this, cut two slices from eggplant, about 1-inch thick, and reserve the remaining eggplant for later use.    Brush slices of eggplant with oil, season with salt on both sides, then Put the slices on grill and cook for 3 to 4 minutes per side.

Move grilled eggplant to a cutting board, let it cool for 5 minutes and then make a home in the center of each slice by using a cookie cutter.    Bring out a frying pan, put it over medium heat, add butter and when it melts, add eggplant slices in it and crack an egg into its each hole. Let the eggs cook, then carefully flip the eggplant slice and continue cooking for 3 minutes until the egg has thoroughly cooked    Season egg with salt and black pepper, move them to a plate, then garnish with green onions and serve.

**Nutrition Info:**184 Cal 14.1 g Fats 7.8 g Protein 3 g Net Carb 3.5 g Fiber

## Breakfast Muffins

Servings: 1    Cooking Time: 5 Minutes
**Ingredients:**
- 1 medium egg
- ¼ cup heavy cream
- 1 slice cooked bacon (cured, pan-fried, cooked)
- 1 oz cheddar cheese
- Salt and black pepper (to taste)

**Directions:**
Preheat the oven to 350°F.    In a bowl, mix the eggs with the cream, salt and pepper.    Spread into muffin tins and fill the cups half full.    Place 1 slice of bacon into each muffin hole and half ounce of cheese on top of each muffin.    Bake for around 15-20 minutes or until slightly browned.    Add another ½ oz of cheese onto each muffin and broil until the cheese is slightly browned. Serve!

**Nutrition Info:**150 cal 11g fat 7g protein 2g carbs

# Meat Recipes

## Stuffed Chicken Breasts Greek-style

Servings: 4    Cooking Time: 20 Minutes

**Ingredients:**
- 4 oz. chicken breasts, skinless and boneless
- ¼ cup onion, minced
- 4 artichoke hearts, minced
- 1 teaspoon oregano, crushed
- 4 lemon slices
- What you will need from the store cupboard:
- 1 cup canned chicken broth, fat-free
- 1-1/2 lemon juice
- 1 tablespoon olive oil
- 2 teaspoons of cornstarch
- Ground pepper
- Salt, optional

**Directions:**
Take out all the fat from the chicken. Wash and pat dry. Season your chicken with pepper and salt.    Pound the chicken to make it flat and thin.    Bring together the oregano, onion, and artichoke hearts.    Now spoon equal amounts of the mix at the center of your chicken. Roll up the log and secure using a skewer or toothpick. Heat oil in your skillet over medium temperature. Add the chicken. Brown all sides evenly.    Pour the lemon juice and broth.    Add lemon slices on top of the chicken. Simmer covered for 10 minutes.    Transfer to a platter. Remove the skewers or toothpick.    Mix cornstarch with a fork.    Transfer to skillet and stir over high temperature.    Put lemon sauce on the chicken.

**Nutrition Info:**Calories 224, Carbohydrates 8g, Fiber 1g, Cholesterol 82mg, Total Fat 5g, Protein 21g, Sodium 339mg

## Shredded Beef

Servings: 2    Cooking Time: 35 Minutes    .

**Ingredients:**
- 1.5lb lean steak
- 1 cup low sodium gravy
- 2tbsp mixed spices

**Directions:**
Mix all the ingredients in your Instant Pot.    Cook on Stew for 35 minutes.    Release the pressure naturally. Shred the beef.

**Nutrition Info:**Calories: 200 Carbs: 2 Sugar: 0 Fat: 5 Protein: 48 GL: 1

## Classic Mini Meatloaf

Servings: 6    Cooking Time: 25 Minutes

**Ingredients:**
- 1 pound 80/20 ground beef
- ¼ medium yellow onion, peeled and diced
- ½ medium green bell pepper, seeded and diced
- 1 large egg
- 3 tablespoons blanched finely ground almond flour
- 1 tablespoon Worcestershire sauce
- ½ teaspoon garlic powder
- 1 teaspoon dried parsley
- 2 tablespoons tomato paste
- ¼ cup water
- 1 tablespoon powdered erythritol

**Directions:**
In a large bowl, combine ground beef, onion, pepper, egg, and almond flour. Pour in the Worcestershire sauce and add the garlic powder and parsley to the bowl. Mix until fully combined.    Divide the mixture into two and place into two (4") loaf baking pans.    In a small bowl, mix the tomato paste, water, and erythritol. Spoon half the mixture over each loaf.    Working in batches if necessary, place loaf pans into the air fryer basket. Adjust the temperature to 350°F and set the timer for 25 minutes or until internal temperature is 180°F.    Serve warm.

**Nutrition Info:**Calories: 170 Protein: 14.9 G Fiber: 0.9 G Net Carbohydrates: 2.6 G Sugar Alcohol: 1.5 G Fat: 9.4 G Sodium: 85 Mg Carbohydrates: 5.0 G Sugar: 1.5 G

## Skirt Steak With Asian Peanut Sauce

Servings: 4    Cooking Time: 15 Minutes

**Ingredients:**
- ⅓ cup light coconut milk
- 1 teaspoon curry powder
- 1 teaspoon coriander powder
- 1 teaspoon reduced-sodium soy sauce
- 1¼ pound skirt steak
- Cooking spray
- ½ cup Asian Peanut Sauce

**Directions:**
In a large bowl, whisk together the coconut milk, curry powder, coriander powder, and soy sauce. Add the steak and turn to coat. Cover the bowl and refrigerate for at least 30 minutes and no longer than 24 hours. Preheat the barbecue or coat a grill pan with cooking spray and place the steak over medium-high heat. Grill the meat until it reaches an internal temperature of 145°F, about 3 minutes per side. Remove the steak from the grill and let it rest for 5 minutes. Slice the steak into 5-ounce pieces and serve each with 2 tablespoons of the Asian Peanut Sauce.    REFRIGERATE: Store the cooled steak in a reseal able container for up to 1 week. Reheat each piece in the microwave for 1 minute.

**Nutrition Info:**Calories: 361 Fat: 22g Saturated Fat: 7g Protein: 36g Total Carbs: 8g Fiber: 2g Sodium: 349mg

## Roasted Pork Loin With Grainy Mustard Sauce

Servings: 8    Cooking Time: 70 Minutes

**Ingredients:**
- 1 (2-pound) boneless pork loin roast
- Sea salt
- Freshly ground black pepper
- 3 tablespoons olive oil

- 1½ cups heavy (whipping) cream
- 3 tablespoons grainy mustard, such as Pommery

**Directions:**

Preheat the oven to 375°F.    Season the pork roast all over with sea salt and pepper.    Place a large skillet over medium-high heat and add the olive oil.    Brown the roast on all sides in the skillet, about 6 minutes in total, and place the roast in a baking dish.    Roast until a meat thermometer inserted in the thickest part of the roast reads 155°F, about 1 hour.    When there is approximately 15 minutes of roasting time left, place a small saucepan over medium heat and add the heavy cream and mustard.    Stir the sauce until it simmers, then reduce the heat to low. Simmer the sauce until it is very rich and thick, about 5 minutes. Remove the pan from the heat and set aside.    Let the pork rest for 10 minutes before slicing and serve with the sauce.

**Nutrition Info:**Calories 368 Fat: 29g Protein: 25g Carbs: 2g Fiber: 0g Net Carbs: 2g Fat 70%/Protein 25%/Carbs 5%

## Meatballs In Tomato Gravy

Servings: 6    Cooking Time: 30 Minutes

**Ingredients:**
- For Meatballs:
- 1 pound lean ground lamb
- 1 tablespoon homemade tomato paste
- ¼ cup fresh cilantro leaves, chopped
- 1 small onion, chopped finely
- 2 garlic cloves, minced
- ½ teaspoon ground cumin
- 1/8 teaspoon salt
- Ground black pepper, as required
- For Tomato Gravy:
- 3 tablespoons olive oil, divided
- 2 medium onions, chopped finely
- 2 garlic cloves, minced
- ½ tablespoon fresh ginger, minced
- 1 teaspoon dried thyme, crushed
- 1 teaspoon dried oregano, crushed
- 3 large tomatoes, chopped finely
- Ground black pepper, as required
- 1½ cups warm low-sodium chicken broth

**Directions:**

For meatballs: in a large bowl, add all the ingredients and mix until well combined.    Make small equal-sized balls from mixture and set aside.    For gravy: in a large pan, heat 1 tablespoon of oil over medium heat.    Add the meatballs and cook for about 4-5 minutes or until lightly browned from all sides.    With a slotted spoon, transfer the meatballs onto a plate.    In the same pan, heat the remaining oil over medium heat and sauté the onion for about 8-10 minutes.    Add the garlic, ginger and herbs and sauté for about 1 minute.    Add the tomatoes and cook for about 3-4 minutes, crushing with the back of spoon.    Add the warm broth and bring to a boil. Carefully, place the meatballs and cook for 5 minutes, without stirring.    Now, reduce the heat to low and cook partially covered for about 15-20 minutes, stirring gently 2-3 times.    Serve hot.    Meal Prep Tip: Transfer the meatballs mixture into a large bowl and set aside to cool.

Divide the mixture into 6 containers evenly. Cover the containers and refrigerate for 1-2 days. Reheat in the microwave before serving.

**Nutrition Info:**Calories 248 Total Fat 12.9 g Saturated Fat 3 g Cholesterol 68 mg Total Carbs 10 g Sugar 4.8 g Fiber 2.5 g Sodium 138 mg Potassium 591 mg Protein 23.4 g

## Garlic-braised Short Rib

Servings: 4    Cooking Time: 2 Hours, 20 Minutes

**Ingredients:**
- 4 (4-ounce) beef short ribs
- Sea salt
- Freshly ground black pepper
- 1 tablespoon olive oil
- 2 teaspoons minced garlic
- ½ cup dry red wine
- 3 cups Rich Beef Stock (here)

**Directions:**

Preheat the oven to 325°F.    Season the beef ribs on all sides with salt and pepper.    Place a deep ovenproof skillet over medium-high heat and add the olive oil. Sear the ribs on all sides until browned, about 6 minutes in total. Transfer the ribs to a plate.    Add the garlic to the skillet and sauté until translucent, about 3 minutes. Whisk in the red wine to deglaze the pan. Be sure to scrape all the browned bits from the meat from the bottom of the pan. Simmer the wine until it is slightly reduced, about 2 minutes.    Add the beef stock, ribs, and any accumulated juices on the plate back to the skillet and bring the liquid to a boil.    Cover the skillet and place it in the oven to braise the ribs until the meat is fall-off-the-bone tender, about 2 hours.    Serve the ribs with a spoonful of the cooking liquid drizzled over each serving.

**Nutrition Info:**Calories: 481 Fat: 38g Protein: 29g Carbs: 5g Fiber: 3g Net Carbs: 2g Fat 70%/Protein 25%/Carbs 5%

## Pulled Pork

Servings: 8    Cooking Time: 2½ Hours

**Ingredients:**
- 2 tablespoons chili powder
- 1 teaspoon garlic powder
- ½ teaspoon onion powder
- ½ teaspoon ground black pepper
- ½ teaspoon cumin

**Directions:**

(4-pound) pork shoulder    In a small bowl, mix chili powder, garlic powder, onion powder, pepper, and cumin. Rub the spice mixture over the pork shoulder, patting it into the skin. Place pork shoulder into the air fryer basket.    Adjust the temperature to 350°F and set the timer for 150 minutes.    Pork skin will be crispy and meat easily shredded with two forks when done. The internal temperature should be at least 145°F.

**Nutrition Info:**Calories: 537 Protein: 42.6 G Fiber: 0.8 G Net Carbohydrates: 0.7 G Fat: 35.5 G Sodium: 180 Mg Carbohydrates: 1.5 G Sugar: 0.2 G

## Rosemary-garlic Lamb Racks

Servings: 4    Cooking Time: 25 Minutes
**Ingredients:**
- 4 tablespoons extra-virgin olive oil
- 2 tablespoons finely chopped fresh rosemary
- 2 teaspoons minced garlic
- Pinch sea salt
- 2 (1-pound) racks French-cut lamb chops (8 bones each)

**Directions:**
In a small bowl, whisk together the olive oil, rosemary, garlic, and salt.    Place the racks in a sealable freezer bag and pour the olive oil mixture into the bag. Massage the meat through the bag so it is coated with the marinade. Press the air out of the bag and seal it. Marinate the lamb racks in the refrigerator for 1 to 2 hours.    Preheat the oven to 450°F.    Place a large ovenproof skillet over medium-high heat. Take the lamb racks out of the bag and sear them in the skillet on all sides, about 5 minutes in total.    Arrange the racks upright in the skillet, with the bones interlaced, and roast them in the oven until they reach your desired doneness, about 20 minutes for medium-rare or until the internal temperature reaches 125°F.    Let the lamb rest for 10 minutes and then cut the racks into chops.    Serve 4 chops per person.
**Nutrition Info:**Calories: 354 Fat: 30g Protein: 21g Carbs: 0g Fiber: 0g Net Carbs: 0g Fat 70%/Protein 30%/Carbs 0%

## Pork Chops In Peach Glaze

Servings: 2    Cooking Time: 16 Minutes
**Ingredients:**
- 2 (6-ounce) boneless pork chops, trimmed
- Sea Salt and ground black pepper, as required
- ½ of ripe yellow peach, peeled, pitted and chopped
- 1 tablespoon olive oil
- 2 tablespoons shallot, minced
- 2 tablespoons garlic, minced
- 2 tablespoons fresh ginger, minced
- 4-6 drops liquid stevia
- 1 tablespoon balsamic vinegar
- ¼ teaspoon red pepper flakes, crushed
- ¼ cup filtered water

**Directions:**
Season the pork chops with sea salt and black pepper generously.    In a blender, add the peach pieces and pulse until a puree forms.    Reserve the remaining peach pieces.    In a skillet, heat the oil over medium heat and sauté the shallots for about 1-2 minutes.    Add the garlic and ginger and sauté for about 1 minute.    Stir in the remaining ingredients and bring to a boil.    Now, reduce the heat to medium-low and simmer for about 4-5 minutes or until a sticky glaze forms.    Remove from the heat and reserve 1/3 of the glaze and set aside. Coat the chops with remaining glaze.    Heat a nonstick skillet over medium-high heat and sear the chops for about 4 minutes per side.    Transfer the chops onto a plate and coat with the remaining glaze evenly.    Serve immediately.    Meal Prep Tip: Transfer the pork chops

into a large bowl and set aside to cool. Divide the chops into 2 containers evenly. Cover the containers and refrigerate for 1-2 days. Reheat in the microwave before serving.
**Nutrition Info:**Calories 359 Total Fat 13.5 g Saturated Fat 3.2 g Cholesterol 124 mg Total Carbs 12 g Sugar 3.8 g Fiber 1.5 g Sodium 102 mg Potassium 938 mg Protein 46.2 g

## Pan Grilled Steak

Servings: 4    Cooking Time: 16 Minutes
**Ingredients:**
- 8 medium garlic cloves, crushed
- 1 (2-inch) piece fresh ginger, sliced thinly
- ¼ cup olive oil
- Salt and ground black pepper, as required
- 1½ pounds flank steak, trimmed

**Directions:**
In a large sealable bag, mix together all ingredients except steak.    Add the steak and coat with marinade generously.    Seal the bag and refrigerate to marinate for about 24 hours.    Remove from refrigerator and keep in room temperature for about 15 minutes. Discard the excess marinade from steak.    Heat a lightly greased grill pan over medium-high heat and cook the steak for about 6-8 minutes per side.    Remove from grill pan and set aside for about 10 minutes before slicing.    With a sharp knife cut into desired slices and serve.    Meal Prep Tip: Transfer the teak slices onto a wire rack to cool completely. With foil pieces, wrap the steak slices and refrigerate for about 1-2 days. Reheat in the microwave before serving.
**Nutrition Info:**Calories 447 Total Fat 26.8 g Saturated Fat 7.7 g Cholesterol 94 mg Total Carbs 2.1g Sugar 0.1 g Fiber 0.2 g Sodium 96 mg Potassium 601 mg Protein 47.7 g

## Air Fryer Beef Empanadas

Servings: 3    Cooking Time: 20 Minutes
**Ingredients:**
- 8 Goya empanada discs, defrosted
- 1 cup picadillo
- 1 egg white, blended
- 1 tsp. water
- Cooking spray

**Directions:**
Set air fryer at 325 degrees F.    Apply a cooking spray to the basket.    Place 2 tbsps. of picadillo to each disc space. Fold in half and secure using a fork. Do the same for all the dough.    Mix water and egg whites. Sprinkle to empanadas top.    Set 3 of them in your air fryer and allow to bake for minutes. Set aside and do the same for the remaining empanadas.
**Nutrition Info:**Calories:183 kcal Carbs: 22g Protein:11 g Fat:5g

## Thyme And Apple Chicken

Servings: 4    Cooking Time: 20 Minutes
**Ingredients:**
- 2 chicken breasts, boneless and skinless

- 1 teaspoon thyme leaves, crushed
- 1 green apple, cored, sliced thin
- 1 shallot, minced
- Thyme sprigs for garnishing
- What you will need from the store cupboard:
- ¼ cup balsamic vinegar
- Salt and pepper to taste
- Cooking spray

**Directions:**
Preheat your oven to 350 °F. Apply cooking spray on your baking dish lightly. Rinse the chicken breasts. Use paper towels to pat dry. Sprinkle salt and pepper on the breasts. Place on your baking dish in a single layer. Keep apple slices around and over the chicken. Sprinkle thyme leaves and shallot. Pour the balsamic vinegar. Bake for 10 minutes. Keep the cooked chicken breasts on a platter. Spoon the cooking juice and apples on top. You can garnish with thyme.
**Nutrition Info:**Calories 163, Carbohydrates 9g, Fiber 1g, Cholesterol 66mg, Total Fat 2g, Protein 27g, Sodium 78mg

## Spiced Leg Of Lamb

Servings: 6     Cooking Time: 1 Hour 40 Minutes
**Ingredients:**
- For Marinade:
- 2/3 cup fat-free plain Greek yogurt
- 1 tablespoon homemade tomato puree
- 1 tablespoon fresh lemon juice
- 3-4 garlic cloves, minced
- 2 tablespoons fresh rosemary, chopped
- 2 teaspoons ground coriander
- 1 teaspoon ground cumin
- 1 teaspoon ground cinnamon
- 1 teaspoon red pepper flakes, crushed
- ¼ teaspoon sweet paprika
- Sea salt and freshly ground black pepper, as required
- 1 (4½-pound) bone-in leg of lamb

**Directions:**
In a large bowl, add yogurt, tomato puree, lemon juice, garlic, rosemary, and spices and mix until well combined. Add leg of lamb and coat with marinade generously. Cover and refrigerate to marinate for about 8-10 hours, flipping occasionally. Remove the marinated leg of lamb from refrigerator and keep in room temperature for about 25-30 minutes before roasting. Preheat the oven to 425 degree F. Line a large roasting pan with a greased foil piece. Arrange the leg of lamb into prepared roasting pan. Roast for 20 minutes. Remove the roasting pan from oven and change the side of leg of lamb. Now, Now, reduce the temperature of oven to 325 degree F. Roast for 40 minutes. Now loosely cover the roasting pan with a large piece of foil. Roast for 40 minutes more. Remove from oven and place onto a cutting board for about 10-15 minutes before slicing. With a sharp knife cut the leg of lamb in desired sized slices and serve. Meal Prep Tip: Transfer the leg slices onto a wire rack to cool completely. With foil pieces, wrap the leg slices and refrigerate for about 1-2 days. Reheat in the microwave before serving.

**Nutrition Info:**Calories 478 Total Fat 15.5 g Saturated Fat 6.1 g Cholesterol 226 mg Total Carbs 3.3 g Sugar 1.3 g Fiber 0.9 g Sodium 226 mg Potassium 48 mg Protein 72.3 g

## Beef With Barley & Veggies

Servings: 2     Cooking Time: 1 Hour 5 Minutes
**Ingredients:**
- ¾ cup filtered water
- ¼ cup pearl barley
- 2 teaspoons olive oil
- 7 ounces lean ground beef
- 1 cup fresh mushrooms, sliced
- ¾ cup onion, chopped
- 2 cups frozen green beans
- ¼ cup low-sodium beef broth
- 2 tablespoon fresh parsley, chopped

**Directions:**
In a pan, add water, barley and pinch of salt and bring to a boil over medium heat. Now, reduce the heat to low and simmer, covered for about 30-40 minutes or until all the liquid is absorbed. Remove from heat and set aside. In a skillet, heat oil over medium-high heat and cook beef for about 8-10 minutes. Add the mushroom and onion and cook f or about 6-7 minutes. Add the green beans and cook for about 2-3 minutes. Stir in cooked barley and broth and cook for about 3-5 minutes more. Stir in the parsley and serve hot. Meal Prep Tip: Transfer the beef mixture into a large bowl and set aside to cool. Divide the mixture into 2 containers evenly. Cover the containers and refrigerate for 1-2 days. Reheat in the microwave before serving.
**Nutrition Info:**Calories 374 Total Fat 11.4 g Saturated Fat 3.1 g Cholesterol 89 mg Total Carbs 32.7g Sugar 1.1 g Fiber 4.2 g Sodium 136 mg Potassium 895 mg Protein 36.6 g

## Taco-stuffed Peppers

Servings: 4     Cooking Time: 15 Minutes
**Ingredients:**
- 1 pound 80/20 ground beef
- 1 tablespoon chili powder
- 2 teaspoons cumin
- 1 teaspoon garlic powder
- 1 teaspoon salt
- ¼ teaspoon ground black pepper
- 1 (10-ounce) can diced tomatoes and green chiles, drained
- 4 medium green bell peppers
- 1 cup shredded Monterey jack cheese, divided

**Directions:**
In a medium skillet over medium heat, brown the ground beef about 7–10 minutes. When no pink remains, drain the fat from the skillet. Return the skillet to the stovetop and add chili powder, cumin, garlic powder, salt, and black pepper. Add drained can of diced tomatoes and chiles to the skillet. Continue cooking 3–5 minutes. While the mixture is cooking, cut each bell pepper in half. Remove the seeds and white membrane. Spoon the cooked mixture evenly into each bell pepper and top with a ¼ cup cheese. Place stuffed peppers into the air fryer

basket. Adjust the temperature to 350°F and set the timer for 15 minutes. When done, peppers will be fork tender and cheese will be browned and bubbling. Serve warm.

**Nutrition Info:**Calories: 346 Protein: 27.8 G Fiber: 3.5 G Net Carbohydrates: 7.2 G Fat: 19.1 G Sodium: 991 Mg Carbohydrates: 10.7 G Sugar: 4.9 G

## Asian Beef Stir-fry

Servings: 4     Cooking Time: 15 Minutes
**Ingredients:**
- ¾ lb. beef top sirloin steak, boneless
- 1/3 teaspoon red pepper, crushed
- ½ red onion, wedges
- 3 cups napa cabbage, shredded
- 2 cups broccoli florets
- What you will need from the store cupboard:
- 3 oz. buckwheat noodles or multigrain spaghetti
- 2 tablespoons teriyaki sauce
- 3 tablespoons orange marmalade, low-sugar
- 2 tablespoons of water
- 2 teaspoons canola oil
- Cooking spray

**Directions:**
Bring together the teriyaki sauce, red pepper, marmalade, and water in a bowl. Keep aside. Cook the spaghetti according to directions on the pack. In the meantime, apply cooking spray on your skillet. Preheat. Now add the red onion and broccoli to your skillet. Cook covered for 3 minutes. Add the carrots and cook for 3 more minutes. The vegetables should become tender. Take out the vegetables. Now add oil and the beef strips. Cook for 3 minutes until the center is slightly pink. Return the vegetables to your skillet with the cabbage and sauce. Cook, while stirring, for 1 minute.

**Nutrition Info:**Calories 279, Carbohydrates 30g, Cholesterol 36mg, Fiber 5g, Sugar 0.8g, Protein 25g, Sodium 259mg

## Pork Loin

Servings: 6     Cooking Time: 20 Minutes
**Ingredients:**
- 1/2 lb. pork tenderloin patted dry
- Non-stick cooking spray
- 2 tbsps. garlic scape pesto
- Salt
- Pepper

**Directions:**
Adjust the temperature of the Air Fryer to 375F. Rub all sides of the tenderloin with the non-stick cooking spray     Add pepper, garlic scape pesto, and salt. Sprinkle the Air Fryer basket with cooking spray. Place the tenderloin on the Air Fryer. Cook the meal at 400°F for 10 minutes. Flip over to the other side and cook for another 10 minutes on the first side. Remove the food from the air fryer. Serve

**Nutrition Info:**Calories: 379 kcal Protein: 8.4g; Fat: 2.2g; Carbs: 0g

## Roasted Pork & Apples

Servings: 4     Cooking Time: 30 Minutes
**Ingredients:**
- Salt and pepper to taste
- ½ teaspoon dried, crushed
- 1 lb. pork tenderloin
- 1 tablespoon canola oil
- 1 onion, sliced into wedges
- 3 cooking apples, sliced into wedges
- ⅔ cup apple cider
- Sprigs fresh sage

**Directions:**
In a bowl, mix salt, pepper and sage. Season both sides of pork with this mixture. Place a pan over medium heat. Brown both sides. Transfer to a roasting pan. Add the onion on top and around the pork. Drizzle oil on top of the pork and apples. Roast in the oven at 425 degrees F for 10 minutes. Add the apples, roast for another 15 minutes. In a pan, boil the apple cider and then simmer for 10 minutes. Pour the apple cider sauce over the pork before serving.

**Nutrition Info:**Calories 239 Total Fat 6 g Saturated Fat 1 g Cholesterol 74 mg Sodium 209 mg Total Carbohydrate 22 g Dietary Fiber 3 g Total Sugars 16 g Protein 24 g Potassium 655 mg

## Nut-stuffed Pork Chops

Servings: 4     Cooking Time: 30 Minutes
**Ingredients:**
- 3 ounces' goat cheese
- ½ cup chopped walnuts
- ¼ cup toasted chopped almonds
- 1 teaspoon chopped fresh thyme
- 4 center-cut pork chops, butterflied
- Sea salt
- Freshly ground black pepper
- 2 tablespoons olive oil

**Directions:**
Preheat the oven to 400°F. In a small bowl, make the filling by stirring together the goat cheese, walnuts, almonds, and thyme until well mixed. Season the pork chops inside and outside with salt and pepper. Stuff each chop, pushing the filling to the bottom of the cut section. Secure the stuffing with toothpicks through the meat. Place a large skillet over medium-high heat and add the olive oil. Pan sear the pork chops until they're browned on each side, about 10 minutes in total. Transfer the pork chops to a baking dish and roast the chops in the oven until cooked through, about 20 minutes. Serve after removing the toothpicks.

**Nutrition Info:**Calories: 481 Fat: 38g Protein: 29g Carbs: 5g Fiber: 3g Net Carbs: 2g Fat 70%/Protein 25%/Carbs 5%

## Braised Lamb With Vegetables

Servings: 6     Cooking Time: 2 Hours And 15 Minutes
**Ingredients:**
- Salt and pepper to taste
- 2 ½ lb. boneless lamb leg, trimmed and sliced into cubes

- 1 tablespoon olive oil
- 1 onion, chopped
- 1 carrot, chopped
- 14 oz. canned diced tomatoes
- 1 cup low-sodium beef broth
- 1 tablespoon fresh rosemary, chopped
- 4 cloves garlic, minced
- 1 cup pearl onions
- 1 cup baby turnips, peeled and sliced into wedges
- 1 ½ cups baby carrots
- 1 ½ cups peas
- 2 tablespoons fresh parsley, chopped

**Directions:**
Sprinkle salt and pepper on both sides of the lamb. Pour oil in a deep skillet. Cook the lamb for 6 minutes. Transfer lamb to a plate. Add onion and carrot. Cook for 3 minutes. Stir in the tomatoes, broth, rosemary and garlic. Simmer for 5 minutes. Add the lamb back to the skillet. Reduce heat to low. Simmer for 1 hour and 15 minutes. Add the pearl onion, baby carrot and baby turnips. Simmer for 30 minutes. Add the peas. Cook for 1 minute. Garnish with parsley before serving.

**Nutrition Info:** Calories 420 Total Fat 14 g Saturated Fat 4 g Cholesterol 126 mg Sodium 529 mg Total Carbohydrate 16 g Dietary Fiber 4 g Total Sugars 7 g Protein 43 g Potassium 988 mg

## Beef With Broccoli

Servings: 4     Cooking Time: 14 Minutes
**Ingredients:**
- 2 tablespoons olive oil, divided
- 2 garlic cloves, minced
- 1 pound beef sirloin steak, trimmed and sliced into thin strips
- ¼ cup low-sodium chicken broth
- 2 teaspoons fresh ginger, grated
- 1 tablespoon ground flax seeds
- ½ teaspoon red pepper flakes, crushed
- Salt and ground black pepper, as required
- 1 large carrot, peeled and sliced thinly
- 2 cups broccoli florets
- 1 medium scallion, sliced thinly

**Directions:**
In a large skillet, heat 1 tablespoon of oil over medium-high heat and sauté the garlic for about 1 minute. Add the beef and cook for about 4-5 minutes or until browned. With a slotted spoon, transfer the beef into a bowl. Remove the excess liquid from skillet. In a bowl, add the broth, ginger, flax seeds, red pepper flakes, salt and black pepper. In the same skillet, heat remaining oil over medium heat. Add the carrot, broccoli and ginger mixture and cook for about 3-4 minutes or until desired doneness. Stir in beef and scallion and cook for about 3-4 minutes. Meal Prep Tip: Transfer the beef mixture into a large bowl and set aside to cool. Divide the mixture into 4 containers evenly. Cover the containers and refrigerate for 1-2 days. Reheat in the microwave before serving.

**Nutrition Info:** Calories 211 Total Fat 14.9 g Saturated Fat 3.9 g Cholesterol 101 mg Total Carbs 6.9 g Sugar 1.9

g Fiber 2.4 g Sodium 108 mg Potassium 706 mg Protein 36.5 g

## Scrambled Eggs With Sausage

Servings: 2     Cooking Time: 10 Minutes
**Ingredients:**
- 2 eggs
- ¼ cup cherry tomatoes
- 1 oz. turkey sausage, cooked and sliced
- 1 whole-grain muffin, halved and toasted
- What you will need from the store cupboard:
- 2 tablespoons chicken broth
- 2 tablespoons low-fat Cheddar cheese, shredded
- Ground black pepper
- Cooking spray

**Directions:**
Apply cooking spray on your skillet. Preheat over medium temperature. Whisk together the broth, black pepper and eggs in a bowl. Stir the sliced sausage in. Now pour in the egg mixture. Cook over medium temperature. Don't stir till you see the mixture starting to set around the edges and at the bottom. Lift the fold the egg mix with a spoon or spatula. The uncooked part should flow below. Keep cooking on medium till it is almost set. Now add the cheese and tomatoes. Cook for a minute more. Serve over the toasted muffin halves.

**Nutrition Info:** Calories 198, Carbohydrates 16g, Fiber 2g, Cholesterol 231mg, Sugar 1g, Fat 9g, Protein 14g

## Carnitas

Servings: 2     Cooking Time: 50 Minutes
**Ingredients:**
- Bay leaves (1)
- Garlic (1 clove slivered)
- Oregano (.25 tsp)
- Garlic powder (.25 tsp)
- Adobo seasoning (.25 tsp.)
- Low-sodium vegetable broth (.25 c)
- Cumin (.5 tsp.)
- Roast (1 lb.)
- Chipotle pepper with adobo sauce (1)

**Directions:**
Set your Instant Pot cooker to sauté. Season the pork as desired before adding it to the Instant Pot cooker and cooking each side for about 5 minutes. Remove the pork from the pot and set aside to cool. With the help of a sharp knife, make a 1-in. incision in the pork that is deep enough to accept the garlic slivers. Add additional seasonings to the pork as desired, rub the mixture into the meat. Add the broth, bay leaf and the chipotle pepper to the Instant Pot before placing it in the Instant Pot cooker pot and sealing the lid of the cooker. Choose the high-pressure option and set the time for 50 minutes. Once the timer goes off, select the instant pressure release option and remove the lid. Remove the pork and shred using a pair of forks. Return the pork to the Instant Pot cooker and allow it to soak up any remaining juices, taking care to remove bay before doing so.

**Nutrition Info:** Protein: 20 grams Carbs: 12.2 grams Fiber: 11.9 grams Sugar: 11.2 grams Fats: 7.5 grams Calories: 320

## Air Fryer Roast Beef

Servings: 3      Cooking Time: 45 Minutes
**Ingredients:**
- 3-1/2 lbs. beef roast
- 2 tbsps. olive oil
- 1 tbsp. rosemary
- 1/2 tbsp. garlic powder
- 1/2 tsp fresh ground rugged black pepper

**Directions:**
Adjust the temperature of the air fryer to 360°F     Mix herbs and oil on a plate. Roll the roast in the blend on the plate to ensure that the entire surface of the beef is covered.     Set the beef in the air fryer basket. Establish the timer for 45 mins for tool-rare beef, 51 mins for the tool. Examine the beef with a meat thermostat to see if it is done to your liking.     Cook for extra 6-minute periods if you like it cooked a lot more. Keep in mind that the roast will undoubtedly remain to prepare while it is relaxing.     Eliminate the roast from the air fryer and put on a plate, cover with lightweight aluminum foil. Allow it to rest for 10 minutes before serving.

**Nutrition Info:** Calories: 666 kcal; Carbs: 0.3g; Fat: 54g; Proteins: 43g

## Pork Chops With Grape Sauce

Servings: 4      Cooking Time: 25 Minutes
**Ingredients:**
- Cooking spray
- 4 pork chops
- ¼ cup onion, sliced
- 1 clove garlic, minced
- ½ cup low-sodium chicken broth
- ¾ cup apple juice
- 1 tablespoon cornstarch
- 1 tablespoon balsamic vinegar
- 1 teaspoon honey
- 1 cup seedless red grapes, sliced in half

**Directions:**
Spray oil on your pan.     Put it over medium heat. Add the pork chops to the pan.     Cook for 5 minutes per side.     Remove and set aside.     Add onion and garlic. Cook for 2 minutes.     Pour in the broth and apple juice. Bring to a boil.     Reduce heat to simmer.     Put the pork chops back to the skillet.     Simmer for 4 minutes. In a bowl, mix the cornstarch, vinegar and honey.     Add to the pan.     Cook until the sauce has thickened.     Add the grapes.     Pour sauce over the pork chops before serving.

**Nutrition Info:** Calories 188 Total Fat 4 g Saturated Fat 1 g Cholesterol 47 mg Sodium 117 mg Total Carbohydrate 18 g Dietary Fiber 1 g Total Sugars 13 g Protein 19 g Potassium 759 mg

## Pork Roast

Servings: 2      Cooking Time: 3 Hours
**Ingredients:**

- Coconut oil (1 T)
- Water (2 c)
- Portobello mushrooms (5 sliced thin)
- Garlic (2 cloves smashed)
- Onion (.5 chopped)
- Celery (1 rib)
- Pepper (.5 tsp.)
- Pork roast (1 lb.)

**Directions:**
Start by adding the garlic onion and celery to the Instant Pot cooker pot before adding in the water and then the roast, before seasoning as desired.     Place the Instant Pot cooker pot into the Instant Pot cooker and seal the lid. Choose the high-pressure option and set the time for 60 minutes.     Once the timer goes off, choose the instant pressure release option     Set the roast aside and place the vegetables and resulting broth into a blender and blend well.     Place the roast back in the Instant Pot cooker, seal the cooker and allow it to cook for 2 hours under high pressure, this will help to render the fat and ensure the edges are crisp.     When the timer goes off, use the instant pressure release option and transfer the roast to a serving dish.     Turn the Instant Pot cooker to the sauté setting before adding in the coconut oil. Once it is heated, add in the mushrooms and allow them to cook for 5 minutes. Add in the gravy from the blender and let it reduce until desired thickness is achieved.     Top roast with gravy prior to serving.

**Nutrition Info:** Protein: 23.8 grams Carbs: 13.2 grams Fiber: 9 grams Sugar: 2.2 grams Fats: 3.5 grams Calories: 360

## Provencal Ribs

Servings: 4      Cooking Time: 20 Minutes
**Ingredients:**
- 500g of pork ribs
- Provencal herbs
- Salt
- Ground pepper
- Oil

**Directions:**
Put the ribs in a bowl and add some oil, Provencal herbs, salt, and ground pepper.     Stir well and leave in the fridge for at least 1 hour.     Put the ribs in the basket of the air fryer and select 2000C for 20 minutes.     From time to time, shake the basket and remove the ribs.

**Nutrition Info:** Calories: 296 kcal Fat: 22.63g Carbs: 0g Protein: 21.71g

## Asparagus Beef Sauté

Servings: 4      Cooking Time: 15 Minutes
**Ingredients:**
- 1 lb. beef tenderloin or sirloin, trimmed and sliced
- 12 oz. asparagus
- 1 carrot, peeled and shredded
- 1 teaspoon crushed herbes de Provence
- ¼ teaspoon lemon peel, grated
- What you will need from the store cupboard:
- ½ cup marsala wine
- 2 teaspoons olive oil
- Cooked rice

- Salt and pepper to taste

**Directions:**
Snap off the asparagus stem ends. Cut into 2-inch pieces. Heat oil over the medium temperature in your skillet. Now cook the carrot, beef, pepper, and salt for 3 minutes. Keep stirring. Add the herbes de Provence and asparagus. Cook for 2 more minutes. Add the lemon peel and marsala. Bring down the heat. Cook for 5 minutes uncovered. Serve with cooked rice.

**Nutrition Info:** Calories 327, Carbohydrates 29g, Fiber 2g, Cholesterol 69mg, Fat 7g, Sugar 0.3g, Protein 28g, Sodium 209mg

## Lamb Leg With Sun-dried Tomato Pesto

Servings: 8     Cooking Time: 70 Minutes

**Ingredients:**
- FOR THE PESTO
- 1 cup sun-dried tomatoes packed in oil, drained
- ¼ cup pine nuts
- 2 tablespoons extra-virgin olive oil
- 2 tablespoons chopped fresh basil
- 2 teaspoons minced garlic
- FOR THE LAMB LEG
- 1 (2-pound) lamb leg
- Sea salt
- Freshly ground black pepper
- 2 tablespoons olive oil

**Directions:**
TO MAKE THE PESTO     Place the sun-dried tomatoes, pine nuts, olive oil, basil, and garlic in a blender or food processor; process until smooth. Set aside until needed. TO MAKE THE LAMB LEG     Preheat the oven to 400°F. Season the lamb leg all over with salt and pepper. Place a large ovenproof skillet over medium-high heat and add the olive oil. Sear the lamb on all sides until nicely browned, about 6 minutes in total. Spread the sun-dried tomato pesto all over the lamb and place the lamb on a baking sheet. Roast until the meat reaches your desired doneness, about 1 hour for medium. Let the lamb rest for 10 minutes before slicing and serving.

**Nutrition Info:** Calories: 352 Fat: 29g Protein: 17g Carbs: 5g Fiber: 2g; Net Carbs: 3g Fat 74%/Protein 20%/Carbs 6%

## Ground Pork With Spinach

Servings: 4     Cooking Time: 15 Minutes

**Ingredients:**
- 1 tablespoon olive oil
- ½ of white onion, chopped
- 2 garlic cloves, chopped finely
- 1 jalapeño pepper, chopped finely
- 1 pound lean ground pork
- 1 teaspoon ground coriander
- 1 teaspoon ground cumin
- ½ teaspoon ground turmeric
- ½ teaspoon ground cinnamon
- ½ teaspoon ground fennel seeds
- Salt and ground black pepper, as required
- ½ cup fresh cherry tomatoes, quartered

- 1¼ pounds collard greens leaves, stemmed and chopped
- 1 teaspoon fresh lemon juice

**Directions:**
In a large skillet, heat the oil over medium heat and sauté the onion for about 4 minutes. Add the garlic and jalapeño pepper and sauté for about 1 minute. Add the pork and spices and cook for about 6 minutes breaking into pieces with the spoon. Stir in the tomatoes and greens and cook, stirring gently for about 4 minutes. Stir in the lemon juice and remove from heat. Serve hot. Meal Prep Tip: Transfer the pork mixture into a large bowl and set aside to cool. Divide the mixture into 4 containers evenly. Cover the containers and refrigerate for 1-2 days. Reheat in the microwave before serving.

**Nutrition Info:** Calories 316 Total Fat 21.8 g Saturated Fat 0.5 g Cholesterol 0 mg Total Carbs 11.4 g Sugar 1.4 g Fiber 5.7 g Sodium 27 mg Potassium 107 mg Protein 23 g

## Vegetable And Egg Muffins

Servings: 6     Cooking Time: 20 Minutes

**Ingredients:**
- 1 tomato, cored, seeded, and chopped
- 2 teaspoons oregano or rosemary, snipped
- ¼ cup onion, chopped
- ¾ cup zucchini, chopped
- 8 eggs
- What you will need from the store cupboard:
- 1 tablespoon olive oil
- ½ cup crumbled feta cheese
- ⅓ cup bulgur
- ⅔ cup of water
- ⅛ teaspoon black pepper, ground
- Cooking spray

**Directions:**
Preheat your oven to 350 °F. Apply cooking spray to the muffin cups. Keep aside. Combine bulgur and water in a saucepan. Boil and then reduce heat. Simmer until the bulgur becomes tender. Drain off the liquid. Cook the onion and zucchini in your skillet over medium temperature. Remove from heat. Stir the cheese, tomato, and bulgur in. Now spoon the mixture into the muffin cups. Whisk together the pepper, oregano, and eggs in a bowl. Pour the vegetable mix in your muffin cups evenly. Bake for 10-12 minutes. Run a knife around the muffin edges to loosen. Remove muffins carefully from the pans. Serve warm.

**Nutrition Info:** Calories 117, Carbohydrates 9g, Fiber 2g, Cholesterol 3mg, Sugar 3g, Protein 11g, Sodium 294mg

## Pork With Bell Peppers

Servings: 4     Cooking Time: 13 Minutes

**Ingredients:**
- 1 tablespoon fresh ginger, chopped finely
- 4 garlic cloves, chopped finely
- 1 cup fresh cilantro, chopped and divided
- ¼ cup plus 1 tablespoon olive oil, divided

- 1 pound tender pork, trimmed, sliced thinly
- 2 onions, sliced thinly
- 1 green bell pepper, seeded and sliced thinly
- 1 red bell pepper, seeded and sliced thinly
- 1 tablespoon fresh lime juice

**Directions:**
In a large bowl, mix together ginger, garlic, ½ cup of cilantro and ¼ cup of oil.    Add the pork and coat with mixture generously.    Refrigerate to marinate for about 2 hours.    Heat a large skillet over medium-high heat and stir fry the pork mixture for about 4-5 minutes. Transfer the pork into a bowl.    In the same skillet, heat remaining oil over medium heat and sauté the onion for about 3 minutes.    Stir in the bell pepper and stir fry for about 3 minutes.    Stir in the pork, lime juice and remaining cilantro and cook for about 2 minutes. Serve hot.    Meal Prep Tip: Transfer the pork mixture into a large bowl and set aside to cool. Divide the mixture into 4 containers evenly. Cover the containers and refrigerate for 1-2 days. Reheat in the microwave before serving.
**Nutrition Info:**Calories 360 Total Fat 21.8 g Saturated Fat 3.9 g Cholesterol 83 mg Total Carbs 11 g Sugar 5.4 g Fiber 2.2 g Sodium 71 mg Potassium 706 mg Protein 31.2 g

### Root Beer Pork

Servings: 2    Cooking Time: 35 Minutes
**Ingredients:**
- Pork roast (1 lb.)
- Black pepper (as desired)
- Onion (.6 c sliced)
- Root beet (.3 c)
- Ketchup (2 T)
- Almond flour (1.5 tsp)
- Lemon juice (.25 tsp) / Worcestershire sauce (1.5 tsp)
- Tomato paste (1 T) / Honey (1.5 tsp)

**Directions:**
Season roast with pepper and garlic salt, and put in the pot.    Mix the rest of the ingredients together and pour on the roast.    Lock and seal the lid.    Set to meat/stew for 35 minutes. Carefully release pressure Take out onions and roast.    Discard the onions and shred the pork.    Stir the pork back into the pot.
**Nutrition Info:**Protein: 19.7grams Carbs: 26.2 grams Fiber: 21.5 grams Sugar: 0 grams Fats: 17.2 grams Calories: 323

### Beef Mushroom Meatballs

Servings: 24 Meatballs    Cooking Time: 30 Minutes
**Ingredients:**
- 1 tablespoon canola or safflower oil
- 1 (8-ounce) container Portobello mushrooms, finely chopped
- Cooking spray
- 1-pound lean ground beef (90% or higher)
- ¾ cup unseasoned bread crumbs
- ½ cup chopped fresh parsley
- 2 garlic cloves, minced
- 1 egg, beaten

- ¼ teaspoon salt
- ⅛ teaspoon freshly ground black pepper

**Directions:**
In a medium skillet over medium heat, heat the oil until it shimmers. Add the mushrooms and sauté until they soften, about 5 minutes. Set aside to slightly cool for 5 minutes.    Preheat the oven to 350°F. Coat a mini muffin tin with the cooking spray.    In a large bowl, combine the mushrooms, beef, bread crumbs, parsley, garlic, egg, salt, and black pepper. Using clean hands, mix until well combined.    Form 1 heaping teaspoon of the beef mixture into a 2-inch ball. Place it into a muffin cup and continue forming meatballs.    Bake until the meatballs are golden brown, about 25 minutes. Let cool for 5 minutes, then use a teaspoon to transfer each meatball into a storage container.    REFRIGERATE: Store the cooled meatballs in a resealable container for up to 1 week. To reheat, microwave for 1 minute. The meatballs also can be reheated in a saucepan over medium heat along with the Speedy Tomato Sauce. FREEZE: Store the cooled meatballs in a freezer-safe container for up to 2 months. Thaw in the refrigerator overnight and reheat in the microwave for 1 minute. The meatballs also can be reheated in a saucepan over medium heat along with the Speedy Tomato Sauce.
**Nutrition Info:**Calories: 232 Fat: 12g Saturated Fat: 4g Protein: 19g Total Carbs: 12g Fiber: 1g Sodium: 276mg

### Pork On A Blanket

Servings: 4    Cooking Time: 10 Minutes
**Ingredients:**
- 1/2 puff defrosted pastry sheet
- 16 thick smoked sausages
- 15 ml of milk

**Directions:**
Adjust the temperature of the air fryer to 200°C and set the timer to 5 minutes.    Cut the puff pastry into 64 x 38 mm strips.    Place a cocktail sausage at the end of the puff pastry and roll around the sausage, sealing the dough with some water.    Brush the top of the sausages wrapped in milk and place them in the preheated air fryer.    Cook at 200°C for 10 minutes or until golden brown.
**Nutrition Info:**Calories: 242 kcal Fat: 14g Carbs: 0g Protein: 27g

### Bacon-wrapped Hot Dog

Servings: 4    Cooking Time: 10 Minutes
**Ingredients:**
- 4 beef hot dogs
- 4 slices sugar-free bacon

**Directions:**
Wrap each hot dog with slice of bacon and secure with toothpick. Place into the air fryer basket.    Adjust the temperature to 370°F and set the timer for 10 minutes. Flip each hot dog halfway through the cooking time. When fully cooked, bacon will be crispy. Serve warm.
**Nutrition Info:**Calories: 197 Protein: 9.2 G Fiber: 0.0 G Net Carbohydrates: 1.3 G Fat: 15.0 G Sodium: 571 Mg Carbohydrates: 1.3 G Sugar: 0.6 G

## Pork Tenderloin

Servings: 6    Cooking Time: 30 Minutes
**Ingredients:**
- 1-1/2 lbs. pork tenderloin

**Directions:**
Adjust the temperature of the Air Fryer to 370F.    Lay the pork in the Air Fryer basket.    Cook at 400F for about 30 minutes, turning halfway through cooking time for a proper cook.    Serve.
**Nutrition Info:**Calories: 419 kcal; Fat: 3.5g; Carbs: 0g; Proteins: 26g

## Bacon Cheeseburger Casserole

Servings: 4    Cooking Time: 20 Minutes
**Ingredients:**
- 1 pound 80/20 ground beef
- ¼ medium white onion, peeled and chopped
- 1 cup shredded Cheddar cheese, divided
- 1 large egg
- 4 slices sugar-free bacon, cooked and crumbled
- 2 pickle spears, chopped

**Directions:**
Brown the ground beef in a medium skillet over medium heat about 7–10 minutes. When no pink remains, drain the fat. Remove from heat and add ground beef to large mixing bowl.    Add onion, ½ cup Cheddar, and egg to bowl. Mix ingredients well and add crumbled bacon. Pour the mixture into a 4-cup round baking dish and top with remaining Cheddar. Place into the air fryer basket. Adjust the temperature to 375°F and set the timer for 20 minutes.    Casserole will be golden on top and firm in the middle when fully cooked. Serve immediately with chopped pickles on top.
**Nutrition Info:**Calories: 369 Protein: 31.0 G Fiber: 0.2 G Net Carbohydrates: 1.0 G Fat: 22.6 G Sodium: 454 Mg Carbohydrates: 1.2 G Sugar: 0.5 G

## Honey Mustard Pork

Servings: 2    Cooking Time: 60 Minutes
**Ingredients:**
- 1.5lb rolled, trimmed pork joint
- 1 cup honey mustard sauce, low carb
- salt and pepper

**Directions:**
Mix all the ingredients in your Instant Pot.    Cook on Stew for 60 minutes.    Release the pressure naturally.
**Nutrition Info:**Calories: 290 Carbs: 9 Sugar: 8 Fat: 17 Protein: 39 GL: 4

## Barbecue Beef Brisket

Servings: 10    Cooking Time: 10 Hours
**Ingredients:**
- 4 lb. beef brisket (boneless), trimmed and sliced
- 1 bay leaf
- 2 onions, sliced into rings
- ½ teaspoon dried thyme, crushed
- ¼ cup chili sauce
- 1 clove garlic, minced
- Salt and pepper to taste
- 2 tablespoons light brown sugar
- 2 tablespoons cornstarch
- 2 tablespoons cold water

**Directions:**
Put the meat in a slow cooker.    Add the bay leaf and onion.    In a bowl, mix the thyme, chili sauce, salt, pepper and sugar.    Pour the sauce over the meat. Mix well.    Seal the pot and cook on low heat for 10 hours.    Discard the bay leaf.    Pour cooking liquid in a pan.    Add the mixed water and cornstarch. Simmer until the sauce has thickened.    Pour the sauce over the meat.
**Nutrition Info:**Calories 182 Total Fat 6 g Saturated Fat 2 g Cholesterol 57 mg Sodium 217 mg Total Carbohydrate 9 g Dietary Fiber 1 g Total Sugars 4 g Protein 20 g Potassium 383 mg

## Cherry Apple Pork

Servings: 2    Cooking Time: 40 Minutes
**Ingredients:**
- Apple (1 small, diced)
- Cherries (.3 c pitted)
- Onion (3 T diced)
- Celery (3 T diced)
- Apple juice (.25 c)
- Black pepper
- Pork loin (.75 lb.)
- Water (.25 c)

**Directions:**
Add all of the ingredients to the Instant Pot cooker and mix thoroughly.    Seal the lid of the cooker, choose the poultry setting and set the time for 5 minutes.    Once the timer goes off, select the quick pressure release option and remove the lid as soon as the pressure has normalized.    Serve warm.
**Nutrition Info:**Protein: 12 grams Carbs: 22.9 grams Fiber: 19 grams Sugar: 11.2 grams Fats: 28 grams Calories: 453

## Italian Sausage Casserole

Servings: 2    Cooking Time: 5 Minutes
**Ingredients:**
- 1lb chopped cooked sausages
- 1lb chopped Mediterranean vegetables
- 1 cup low sodium broth
- 1tbsp mixed herbs

**Directions:**
Mix all the ingredients in your Instant Pot.    Cook on Stew for 5 minutes.    Release the pressure naturally.
**Nutrition Info:**Calories: 320 Carbs: 8 Sugar: 2 Fat: 18 Protein: 41 GL: 4

## Pork Fillets With Serrano Ham

Servings: 4    Cooking Time: 20 Minutes
**Ingredients:**
- 400g of very thin sliced pork fillets
- 2 boiled and chopped eggs
- 100g chopped Serrano ham
- 1 beaten egg
- Breadcrumbs

**Directions:**

Make a roll with the pork fillets. Introduce half-cooked egg and Serrano ham. So that the roll does not lose its shape, fasten with a string or chopsticks. Pass the rolls through the beaten egg and then through the breadcrumbs until it forms a good layer. Adjust the temperature of the air fryer for a few minutes at 180° C. Insert the rolls in the basket and set the timer for about 8 minutes at 180° C. Serve.
**Nutrition Info:**Calories: 424 kcal Fat: 15.15g Carbs: 37.47g Protein: 31.84g

## Maple Glazed Pork

Servings: 2    Cooking Time: 15 Minutes
**Ingredients:**
- Maple syrup (.25 c)
- Honey (.25 c)
- Cinnamon (1 tsp)
- Brown sugar (.25 c)
- Orange juice (2 T)
- Nutmeg (1 tsp)
- Bone in ham (1 small)

**Directions:**
Combine everything except for the ham in a saucepan on medium heat; mix well. Put the ham in the cooker. Cook 15 minutes, then use quick release. Set the ham in the baking dish. Pour glaze over ham. Place the ham under a broiler to caramelize the sugars and form a slight char.
**Nutrition Info:**Protein: 23.8 grams Carbs: 37.5 grams Fiber: 32.8 grams Sugar: 18.2 grams Fats: 42 grams Calories: 540

## Grilled Chicken Wraps

Servings: 4    Cooking Time: 6 Minutes
**Ingredients:**
- 4 oz. chicken breasts, boneless and skinless
- 2 teaspoons oregano, crushed
- ¼ cup mint, chopped
- 2 onion slices, peeled
- What you will need from the store cupboard:
- 2 12-inch Arabic bread or Naan pieces
- 2 tablespoons of lemon juice
- Cooking spray
- Pepper and salt to taste

**Directions:**
Preheat your oven to 350 °F. Brush both sides of the chicken breasts with lemon juice. Sprinkle oregano. Apply cooking spray lightly and return to the grill. Keep the onion slices and chicken breasts on the grill. Cook each side for 3 minutes. Turn once. Cut the onion into strips. Cut the chicken into small ½ strips after it is done. Cut your Arabic bread into half. Leave the pita bread or naan whole. Now keep the onion strips and chicken at the center of the bread pieces. Sprinkle mint. Roll up.
**Nutrition Info:**Calories 328, Carbohydrates 36g, Fiber 5g, Cholesterol 82mg, Total Fat 3g, Protein 39g, Sodium 415mg

## Sirloin With Blue Cheese Compound Butter

Servings: 4    Cooking Time: 12 Minutes
**Ingredients:**
- 6 tablespoons butter, at room temperature
- 4 ounces' blue cheese, such as Stilton or Roquefort
- 4 (5-ounce) beef sirloin steaks
- 1 tablespoon olive oil
- Sea salt
- Freshly ground black pepper

**Directions:**
Place the butter in a blender and pulse until the butter is whipped, about 2 minutes. Add the cheese and pulse until just incorporated. Spoon the butter mixture onto a sheet of plastic wrap and roll it into a log about 1½ inches in diameter by twisting both ends of the plastic wrap in opposite directions. Refrigerate the butter until completely set, about 1 hour. Slice the butter into ½-inch disks and set them on a plate in the refrigerator until you are ready to serve the steaks. Store leftover butter in the refrigerator for up to 1 week. Preheat a barbecue to medium-high heat. Let the steaks come to room temperature. Rub the steaks all over with the olive oil and season them with salt and pepper. Grill the steaks until they reach your desired doneness, about 6 minutes per side for medium. If you do not have a barbecue, broil the steaks in a preheated oven for 7 minutes per side for medium. Let the steaks rest for 10 minutes. Serve each topped with a disk of the compound butter.
**Nutrition Info:**Calories: 544 Fat: 44g Protein: 35g Carbs: 0g Fiber: 0g Net Carbs: 0g Fat 72%/Protein 28%/Carbs 0%

## Pork Rind

Servings: 4    Cooking Time: 1 Hr
**Ingredients:**
- 1kg pork rinds
- Salt
- 1/2 tsp black pepper coffee

**Directions:**
Preheat the air fryer. Set the time of 5 minutes and the temperature to 2000C. Cut the bacon into cubes - 1 finger wide. Season with salt and a pinch of pepper. Place in the basket of the air fryer. Set the time of 45 minutes and press the power button. Shake the basket every 10 minutes so that the pork rinds stay golden brown equally. Once they are ready, drain a little on the paper towel, so they stay dry. Transfer to a plate and serve.
**Nutrition Info:**Calories: 172 kcal Fat: 10.02g Carbs: 0g Protein: 19.62g

## Roasted Pork Shoulder

Servings: 12    Cooking Time: 6 Hours
**Ingredients:**
- 1 head garlic, peeled and crushed
- ¼ cup fresh rosemary, minced
- 2 tablespoons fresh lemon juice
- 2 tablespoons balsamic vinegar
- 1 (4-pound) pork shoulder, trimmed

**Directions:**
In a bowl, add all the ingredients except pork shoulder and mix well.    In a large roasting pan place pork shoulder and coat with marinade generously.    With a large plastic wrap, cover the roasting pan and refrigerate to marinate for at least 1-2 hours.    Remove the roasting pan from refrigerator.    Remove the plastic wrap from roasting pan and keep in room temperature for 1 hour.    Preheat the oven to 275 degrees F. Arrange the roasting pan in oven and roast for about 6 hours.    Remove from the oven and set aside for about 15-20 minutes.    With a sharp knife, cut the pork shoulder into desired slices and serve.    Meal Prep Tip: Transfer the pork slices onto a wire rack to cool completely. With foil pieces, wrap the pork slices and refrigerate for about 1-2 days. Reheat in the microwave before serving.
**Nutrition Info:**Calories 450 Total Fat 32.6g Saturated Fat 12 g Cholesterol 136 mg Total Carbs 1.5 g Sugar 0.1 g Fiber 0.6 g Sodium 104 mg Potassium 522 mg Protein 35.4 g

## Lamb Curry

Servings: 8      Cooking Time: 2¼ Hours
**Ingredients:**
- For Spice Mixture:
- 2 teaspoons ground coriander
- 2 teaspoons ground cumin
- 1 teaspoon ground cinnamon
- ½ teaspoon ground ginger
- 1 tablespoons sweet paprika
- ½ tablespoon cayenne pepper
- 1 teaspoon red chili powder
- Salt and ground black pepper, as required
- For Curry:
- 1 tablespoon olive oil
- 2 pounds boneless lamb, trimmed and cubed into 1-inch size
- 2 cups onions, chopped
- ½ cup fat-free plain Greek yogurt, whipped
- 1½ cups water

**Directions:**
For spice mixture: in a bowl, add all spices and mix well. Set aside.    In a large Dutch oven, heat the oil over medium-high heat and stir fry the lamb cubes for about 5 minutes.    Add the onion and cook for about 4-5 minutes.    Stir in the spice mixture and cook for about 1 minute.    Add the yogurt and water and bring to a boil over high heat.    Now, reduce the heat to low and simmer, covered for about 1-2 hours or until desired doneness of lamb.    Uncover and simmer for about 3-4 minutes.    Serve hot.    Meal Prep Tip: Transfer the curry into a large bowl and set aside to cool. Divide the curry into 8 containers evenly. Cover the containers and refrigerate for 1-2 days. Reheat in the microwave before serving.
**Nutrition Info:**Calories 254 Total Fat 10.5 g Saturated Fat 3.3 g Cholesterol 102 mg Total Carbs 4.7 g Sugar 1.9 g Fiber 1.4 g Sodium 99 mg Potassium 468 mg Protein 34 g

## Mediterranean Lamb Meatballs

Servings: 8      Cooking Time: 20 Minutes
**Ingredients:**
- 12 oz. roasted red peppers
- 1 ½ cups whole wheat breadcrumbs
- 2 eggs, beaten
- 1/3 cup tomato sauce
- ½ cup fresh basil
- ¼ cup parsley, snipped
- Salt and pepper to taste
- 2 lb. lean ground lamb

**Directions:**
Preheat your oven to 350 degrees F.    In a bowl, mix all the ingredients and then form into meatballs.    Put the meatballs on a baking pan.    Bake in the oven for 20 minutes.
**Nutrition Info:**Calories 94 Total Fat 3 g Saturated Fat 1 g Cholesterol 35 mg Sodium 170 mg Total Carbohydrate 2 g Dietary Fiber 1 g Total Sugars 0 g Protein 14 g Potassium 266 mg

## Irish Pork Roast

Servings: 8      Cooking Time: 1 Hour
**Ingredients:**
- 1 ½ lb. parsnips, peeled and sliced into small pieces
- 1 ½ lb. carrots, sliced into small pieces
- 3 tablespoons olive oil, divided
- 2 teaspoons fresh thyme leaves, divided
- Salt and pepper to taste
- 2 lb. pork loin roast
- 1 teaspoon honey
- 1 cup dry hard cider
- Applesauce

**Directions:**
Preheat your oven to 400 degrees F.    Drizzle half of the oil over the parsnips and carrots.    Season with half of thyme, salt and pepper.    Arrange on a roasting pan. Rub the pork with the remaining oil.    Season with the remaining thyme.    Season with salt and pepper. Put it on the roasting pan on top of the vegetables. Roast for 65 minutes.    Let cool before slicing. Transfer the carrots and parsnips in a bowl and mix with honey.    Add the cider.    Place in a pan and simmer over low heat until the sauce has thickened.    Serve the pork with the vegetables and applesauce.
**Nutrition Info:**Calories 272 Total Fat 8 g Saturated Fat 2 g Cholesterol 61 mg Sodium 327 mg Total Carbohydrate 23 g Dietary Fiber 6 g Total Sugars 10 g Protein 24 g Potassium 887 mg

## Vegetables With Irish Beef Roast

Servings: 8      Cooking Time: 20 Minutes
**Ingredients:**
- 1 beef rump roast, boneless
- 2 packs mushrooms
- 2 packs (each 1.5 lb.) pot roast vegetables – onions, potatoes, celery, carrots
- 1/3 cup parsley, chopped
- What you will need from the store cupboard:

- 1/3 cup all-purpose flour
- 1 cup beer
- ½ teaspoon black pepper
- ½ teaspoon salt

**Directions:**
Cut the potatoes in half, celery and carrots into 2-inch pieces, and the onions into half-inch wedges. Keep aside. Bring together the gravy mixes, salt, pepper, and flour in a bowl. Now add the vegetables to this bowl. Toss for coating. Take out all vegetables form the flour mix. Keep in a cooker. Add the beef roast to bowl. Coat with the flour mixture evenly. Take out the roast. Keep in the cooker at the center of your vegetables. Now whisk the beer into the remaining flour mix until it is smooth. Add to the cooker. Cook covered. Remove the vegetables and roast. Skim fat from the gravy. Create thin slices from the roast. Serve with gravy and vegetables. If you want, you can sprinkle parsley.
**Nutrition Info:**Calories 318, Carbohydrates 17g, Cholesterol 112mg, Fat 9g, Fiber 3g, Protein 39g, Sodium 516mg

## Rosemary Lamb

Servings: 14     Cooking Time: 2 Hours
**Ingredients:**
- Salt and pepper to taste
- 2 teaspoons fresh rosemary, snipped
- 5 lb. whole leg of lamb, trimmed and cut with slits on all sides
- 3 cloves garlic, slivered
- 1 cup water

**Directions:**
Preheat your oven to 375 degrees F. Mix salt, pepper and rosemary in a bowl. Sprinkle mixture all over the lamb. Insert slivers of garlic into the slits. Put the lamb on a roasting pan. Add water to the pan. Roast for 2 hours.
**Nutrition Info:**Calories 136 Total Fat 4 g Saturated Fat 1 g Cholesterol 71 mg Sodium 218 mg Protein 23 g Potassium 248 mg

## Roast Pork

Servings: 6     Cooking Time: 30 Minutes
**Ingredients:**
- 2 lbs. pork loin
- 1 Tbsp. olive oil
- 1 tsp. salt

**Directions:**
Adjust the temperature of the Air Fryer to 360F. Apply the oil on the pork. Add salt. Cook the pork in the Air Fryer for about 50 minutes. Shake the food halfway through the cooking Remove the meal from Air Fryer and allow it to cool. Serve
**Nutrition Info:**Calories: 150 kcal Fat: 6g; Carbs: 0g; Protein: 23.1g

## Marinated Loin Potatoes

Servings: 4     Cooking Time: 1 Hr
**Ingredients:**
- 2 medium potatoes

- 4 fillets of marinated loin
- A little extra virgin olive oil
- Salt

**Directions:**
Peel the potatoes and cut. Cut with match-sized mandolin, potatoes with a cane but very thin. Wash and immerse in water 30 minutes. Drain and dry well. Add a little oil and stir so that the oil permeates well in all the potatoes. Go to the basket of the air fryer and distribute well. Cook at 1600C for 10 minutes. Take out the basket, shake so that the potatoes take off. Let the potato tender. If it is not, leave 5 more minutes. Place the steaks on top of the potatoes. Select, 10 minutes, and 1800C for 5 minutes again.
**Nutrition Info:**Calories: 136 kcal Fat: 5.1g Carbs: 1.9g Protein: 20.7g

## Curried Lamb On Rice

Servings: 4     Cooking Time: 20 Minutes
**Ingredients:**
- 1 lb. lean lamb, trimmed and cubed
- ¼ teaspoon ginger, ground
- 1 tomato, peeled, seeded and chopped
- ½ cup carrot, grated
- ½ cup onion, chopped
- What you will need from the store cupboard:
- 2 cups of cooked rice
- 1 cup beef broth
- 1 tablespoon margarine
- ¾ teaspoon salt
- 2 teaspoons of curry powder
- 1-1/2 tablespoons all-purpose flour

**Directions:**
Heat a skillet and brown the onion and lamb for 5 minutes in the margarine. Add the curry powder, broth, flour, tomato, and salt. Mix well by stirring. Simmer until the lamb has become tender. Add some water and keep stirring. Now toss the carrot with your rice in a saucepan. Heat. Divide your rice among the serving plates. Place lamb over the rice.
**Nutrition Info:**Calories 331, Carbohydrates 31g, Fiber 2g, Cholesterol 75mg, Fat 10g, Protein 28g, Sugar 1g

## Pork With Pear Stuffing

Servings: 4     Cooking Time: 20 Minutes
**Ingredients:**
- 1 pork tenderloin
- ¼ cup carrot, shredded
- ½ cup pear, chopped
- 2 tablespoons onion, chopped
- ½ cup pear, chopped
- What you will need from the store cupboard:
- 1 teaspoon cooking oil
- ¼ cup soft breadcrumbs
- 2 tablespoons orange marmalade, sugar-free
- ¼ teaspoon pepper
- ¼ teaspoon salt

**Directions:**
For the stuffing, bring together the breadcrumbs, pear, onion, pepper, and salt in a bowl. Keep this aside. Trim fat from the meat. Cut lengthwise down the center.

Open flat. Pound the flat side.    Now spread stuffing over your meat. Fold in the ends. Roll up.    Use wooden toothpicks or kitchen string to secure.    Keep meat roll in your roasting pan.    Brush oil lightly.    Roast for 12 minutes.    Brush some orange marmalade over the meat's top.    Roast again for 3 minutes.

**Nutrition Info:**Calories 191, Carbohydrates 9g, Fiber 2g, Cholesterol 55mg, Fat 9g, Sugar 0.3g, Protein 20g, Sodium 193mg

## Pork Curry

Servings: 2     Cooking Time: 20 Minutes

**Ingredients:**

- Carrots (2 sliced)
- Turmeric (.25 tsp.)
- Garam masala (1.5 T)
- Diced tomatoes (4 oz.)
- Zucchini (.25 diced)
- Ghee (1 T)
- Black pepper (1 pinch)
- Coconut milk (.5 c)
- Onion (.5 diced)
- Lime juice (.5 limes)
- Ginger (1 inch grated)
- Garlic (2 cloves minced)
- Pork (1 lb.)

**Directions:**

In a sealable container, place the meat before adding in the coconut milk, garlic, lime juice and ginger and mixing thoroughly. Allow the meat to marinate overnight for best results.    Place the onions, carrots, garam masala, ghee, tomatoes and meat together in the Instant Pot cooker pot and combine thoroughly.    Place the Instant Pot cooker pot into the Instant Pot cooker and seal the lid. Choose the high-pressure option and set the time for 20 minutes.    Once the timer goes off, select the natural pressure release option and allow the pot to sit for 10 minutes    After opening the lid, switch the Instant Pot cooker to sauté before adding in the zucchini and letting it simmer for 5 minutes.    Serve hot over shirataki rice.

**Nutrition Info:**Protein: 38 grams Carbs: 29 grams Fiber: 23 grams Sugar: 3.5 grams Fats: 33 grams Calories: 520

## Lamb Chops With Kalamata Tapenade

Servings: 4     Cooking Time: 25 Minutes

**Ingredients:**

- FOR THE TAPENADE
- 1 cup pitted Kalamata olives
- 2 tablespoons chopped fresh parsley
- 2 tablespoons extra-virgin olive oil
- 2 teaspoons minced garlic
- 2 teaspoons freshly squeezed lemon juice
- FOR THE LAMB CHOPS
- 2 (1-pound) racks French-cut lamb chops (8 bones each)
- Sea salt
- Freshly ground black pepper
- 1 tablespoon olive oil

**Directions:**

Place the olives, parsley, olive oil, garlic, and lemon juice in a food processor and process until the mixture is puréed but still slightly chunky.    Transfer the tapenade to a container and store sealed in the refrigerator until needed.    TO MAKE THE LAMB CHOPS    Preheat the oven to 450°F.    Season the lamb racks with salt and pepper.    Place a large ovenproof skillet over medium-high heat and add the olive oil.    Pan sear the lamb racks on all sides until browned, about 5 minutes in total.    Arrange the racks upright in the skillet, with the bones interlaced, and roast them in the oven until they reach your desired doneness, about 20 minutes for medium-rare or until the internal temperature reaches 125°F.    Let the lamb rest for 10 minutes and then cut the lamb racks into chops. Arrange 4 chops per person on the plate and top with the Kalamata tapenade.

**Nutrition Info:**Calories: 348 Fat: 28g Protein: 21g Carbs: 2g Fiber: 1g Net Carbs: 1g Fat 72%/Protein 25%/Carbs 3%

## Chicken With Asparagus And Mango

Servings: 4     Cooking Time: 15 Minutes

**Ingredients:**

- 1 lb. chicken breast, skinless
- 1 ripe mango, peeled, cut into chunks
- 6 oz. asparagus, cut into 2-inch pieces
- 1 egg white
- ½ red bell pepper, seeded
- What you will need from the store cupboard:
- ½ tablespoon canola oil
- 2-1/2 tablespoons vodka
- ½ cup dry white wine
- 1 tablespoon of cornstarch
- 1 tablespoon soy sauce, low-sodium

**Directions:**

Keep the chicken in a bowl.    Now add the cornstarch, egg white, canola oil, and vodka. Stir to coat well.    Set aside, while preparing the other part of the recipe. Bring together the soy sauce, chicken stock and white wine in your pitcher.    Heat your nonstick skillet. Apply cooking oil.    Add your marinated chicken. Cook over high temperature until it browns.    Add the asparagus and red pepper. Stir fry for 1 minute.    Stir the liquid in slowly. Boil to thicken the sauce.    Bring down the heat. Stir the mango in.    Serve with basmati rice.

**Nutrition Info:**Calories 213, Carbohydrates 9g, Fiber 2g, Cholesterol 66mg, Total Fat 3g, Protein 29g, Sodium 231mg

## Steak With Mushroom Sauce

Servings: 4     Cooking Time: 5 Minutes

**Ingredients:**

- 12 oz. sirloin steak, sliced and trimmed
- 2 teaspoons grilling seasoning
- 2 teaspoons oil
- 6 oz. broccoli, trimmed
- 2 cups frozen peas
- 3 cups fresh mushrooms, sliced
- 1 cup beef broth (unsalted)
- 1 tablespoon mustard
- 2 teaspoons cornstarch

- Salt to taste

**Directions:**
Preheat your oven to 350 degrees F.    Season meat with grilling seasoning.    In a pan over medium high heat, cook the meat and broccoli for 4 minutes.    Sprinkle the peas around the steak.    Put the pan inside the oven and bake for 8 minutes.    Remove both meat and vegetables from the pan.    Add the mushrooms to the pan.    Cook for 3 minutes.    Mix the broth, mustard, salt and cornstarch.    Add to the mushrooms.    Cook for 1 minute.    Pour sauce over meat and vegetables before serving.

**Nutrition Info:**Calories 226 Total Fat 6 g Saturated Fat 2 g Cholesterol 51 mg Sodium 356 mg Total Carbohydrate 16 g Dietary Fiber 5 g Total Sugars 6 g Protein 26 g Potassium 780 mg

## Air Fryer Bacon

Servings: 4     Cooking Time: 10 Minutes
**Ingredients:**
- 11 slices bacon

**Directions:**
Divide the bacon in half, and place the first half in the air fryer.    Set the temperature at 401 degrees F, and set the timer to 11 mins.    Check it halfway through to see if anything needs to be rearranged.    Cook remainder of the time. Serve.

**Nutrition Info:**Calories: 91 kcal Carbs: 0g Protein: 2g Fat: 8g

## Chorizo And Beef Burger

Servings: 4     Cooking Time: 15 Minutes
**Ingredients:**
- ¾ pound 80/20 ground beef
- ¼ pound Mexican-style ground chorizo
- ¼ cup chopped onion
- 5 slices pickled jalapeños, chopped
- 2 teaspoons chili powder
- 1 teaspoon minced garlic
- ¼ teaspoon cumin

**Directions:**

In a large bowl, mix all ingredients. Divide the mixture into four sections and form them into burger patties. Place burger patties into the air fryer basket, working in batches if necessary.    Adjust the temperature to 375°F and set the timer for 15 minutes.    Flip the patties halfway through the cooking time. Serve warm.

**Nutrition Info:**Calories: 291 Protein: 21.6 G Fiber: 0.9 G Net Carbohydrates: 3.8 G Fat: 18.3 G Sodium: 474 Mg Carbohydrates: 4.7 G Sugar: 2.5 G

## Lamb & Chickpeas

Servings: 4     Cooking Time: 30 Minutes
**Ingredients:**
- 1 lb. lamb leg (boneless), trimmed and sliced into small pieces
- 2 tablespoons olive oil
- 1 teaspoon ground coriander
- Salt and pepper to taste
- ½ teaspoon ground cumin
- ¼ teaspoon red pepper, crushed
- ¼ cup fresh mint, chopped
- 2 teaspoons lemon zest
- 2 cloves garlic, minced
- 30 oz. unsalted chickpeas, rinsed and drained
- 1 cup tomatoes, chopped
- 1 cup English cucumber, chopped
- ¼ cup fresh parsley, snipped
- 1 tablespoon red wine vinegar

**Directions:**
Preheat your oven to 375 degrees F.    Place the lamb on a baking dish.    Toss in half of the following: oil, cumin and coriander.    Season with red pepper, salt and pepper.    Mix well.    Roast for 20 minutes.    In a bowl, combine the rest of the ingredients with the remaining seasonings.    Add salt and pepper.    Serve lamb with chickpea mixture.

**Nutrition Info:**Calories 366 Total Fat 15 g Saturated Fat 3 g Cholesterol 74 mg Sodium 369 mg Total Carbohydrate 27 g Dietary Fiber 7 g Total Sugars 3 g Protein 32 g Potassium 579 mg

# Poultry Recipes

## Crunchy Chicken Fingers

Servings: 2    Cooking Time: 4 Minutes

**Ingredients:**
- 2 medium-sized chicken breasts, cut in stripes
- 3 tbsp parmesan cheese
- ¼ tbsp fresh chives, chopped
- ⅓ cup breadcrumbs
- 1 egg white
- 2 tbsp plum sauce, optional
- ½ tbsp fresh thyme, chopped
- ½ tbsp black pepper
- 1 tbsp water

**Directions:**
Preheat the Air Fryer to 360 F. Mix the chives, parmesan, thyme, pepper and breadcrumbs. In another bowl, whisk the egg white and mix with the water. Dip the chicken strips into the egg mixture and the breadcrumb mixture. Place the strips in the air fryer basket and cook for 10 minutes. Serve with plum sauce.

**Nutrition Info:**Calories: 253; Carbs: 31g; Fat: 18g; Protein: 28g

## Polynesian Chicken

Servings: 6 Cups    Cooking Time: 4 Hours

**Ingredients:**
- 3 garlic cloves, minced
- 2 bell peppers, cut into 1/2-inch strips
- 1 (20-ounce) can pineapple chunks in juice, drained, with juice reserved
- 1 1/2-pound boneless chicken breasts, cut into 2-inch cubes
- 1/3 cup honey
- 2 tablespoons tapioca flour
- 3 tablespoons low-sodium soy sauce
- 1 teaspoon ground ginger

**Directions:**
Add reserved pineapple juice, 3 tablespoons of soy sauce, 1/3 cup honey, 1 teaspoon ground ginger and 3 minced cloves of garlic into a bowl; whisk well. Then add 2 tablespoons tapioca flour and whisk again until combined.    Add chicken along with chunks of pineapple into a slow cooker.    Pour mixture of pineapple juice over chicken and cover the cooker. Cook for about 4-5 hours on low, until chicken is completely cooked through.    Then add strips of bell pepper in the last hour of cooking. Serve and enjoy!

**Nutrition Info:**273 calories; 26 g fat; 37 g total carbs; 26 g protein

## Buffalo Chicken

Servings: 8    Cooking Time: 30 Minutes

**Ingredients:**
- 2 celery stalks, diced
- 1 medium-sized onion, chopped
- 100 ml buffalo wing sauce
- 100 ml chicken broth
- 21 kg chicken breasts, frozen

**Directions:**
Add the celery, onions, wing sauce, chicken broth and chicken to the Instant Pot. Cook frozen chicken on high pressure for 20 minutes. Turn the pressure valve to "Vent" to release all of the pressure.    Remove the chicken breasts from the pot, and shred.    You can remove most of the liquid from the pot, or not.

**Nutrition Info:**Calories: 197 Fat: 8g Carbohydrates: 16g Protein: 14g

## Chicken & Peanut Stir-fry

Servings: 4    Cooking Time: 15 Minutes

**Ingredients:**
- 3 tablespoons lime juice
- ½ teaspoon lime zest
- 4 cloves garlic, minced
- 2 teaspoons chili bean sauce
- 1 tablespoon fish sauce
- 1 tablespoon water
- 2 tablespoons peanut butter
- 3 teaspoons oil, divided
- 1 lb. chicken breast, sliced into strips
- 1 red sweet pepper, sliced into strips
- 3 green onions, sliced thinly
- 2 cups broccoli, shredded
- 2 tablespoons peanuts, chopped

**Directions:**
In a bowl, mix the lime juice, lime zest, garlic, chili bean sauce, fish sauce, water and peanut butter.    Mix well. In a pan over medium high heat, add 2 teaspoons of oil. Cook the chicken until golden on both sides.    Pour in the remaining oil.    Add the pepper and green onions. Add the chicken, broccoli and sauce.    Cook for 2 minutes.    Top with peanuts before serving.

**Nutrition Info:**Calories 368 Total Fat 11 g Saturated Fat 2 g Cholesterol 66 mg Sodium 556 mg Total Carbohydrate 34 g Dietary Fiber 3 g Total Sugars 4 g Protein 32 g Potassium 482 mg

## Meatballs Curry

Servings: 6    Cooking Time: 25 Minutes

**Ingredients:**
- For Meatballs:
- 1 pound lean ground chicken
- 1 tablespoon onion paste
- 1 teaspoons fresh ginger paste
- 1 teaspoons garlic paste
- 1 green chili, chopped finely
- 1 tablespoon fresh cilantro leaves, chopped
- 1 teaspoon ground coriander
- ½ teaspoon cumin seeds
- ½ teaspoon red chili powder
- ½ teaspoon ground turmeric
- 1/8 teaspoon salt
- For Curry:
- 3 tablespoons olive oil
- ½ teaspoon cumin seeds

- 1 (1-inch) cinnamon stick
- 2 onions, chopped
- 1 teaspoons fresh ginger, minced
- 1 teaspoons garlic, minced
- 4 tomatoes, chopped finely
- 2 teaspoons ground coriander
- 1 teaspoon garam masala powder
- ½ teaspoon ground nutmeg
- ½ teaspoon red chili powder
- ½ teaspoon ground turmeric
- Salt, as required
- 1 cup filtered water
- 3 tablespoons fresh cilantro, chopped

**Directions:**
For meatballs: in a large bowl, add all ingredients and mix until well combined.     Make small equal-sized meatballs from mixture.     In a large deep skillet, heat the oil over medium heat and cook the meatballs for about 3-5 minutes or until browned from all sides. Transfer the meatballs into a bowl.     In the same skillet, add the cumin seeds and cinnamon stick and sauté for about 1 minute.     Add the onions and sauté for about 4-5 minutes.     Add the ginger and garlic paste and sauté for about 1 minute.     Add the tomato and spices and cook, crushing with the back of spoon for about 2-3 minutes.     Add the water and meatballs and bring to a boil.     Now, reduce the heat to low and simmer for about 10 minutes.     Serve hot with the garnishing of cilantro.     Meal Prep Tip: Transfer the curry into a large bowl and set aside to cool. Divide the curry into 5 containers evenly. Cover the containers and refrigerate for 1-2 days. Reheat in the microwave before serving.
**Nutrition Info:**Calories 196 Total Fat 11.4 g Saturated Fat 2.4 g Cholesterol 53 mg Total Carbs 7.9 g Sugar 3.9 g Fiber 2.1 g Sodium 143 mg Potassium 279 mg Protein 16.7 g

### Jerk Style Chicken Wings

Servings: 2-3     Cooking Time: 25 Minutes.
**Ingredients:**
- 1g ground thyme
- 1g dried rosemary
- 2g allspice
- 4g ground ginger
- 3 g garlic powder
- 2g onion powder
- 1g of cinnamon
- 2g of paprika
- 2g chili powder
- 1g nutmeg
- Salt to taste
- 30 ml of vegetable oil
- 0.5 - 1 kg of chicken wings
- 1 lime, juice

**Directions:**
Select Preheat, set the temperature to 200°C and press Start/Pause.     Combine all spices and oil in a bowl to create a marinade.     Mix the chicken wings in the marinade until they are well covered.     Place the chicken wings in the preheated air fryer.     Select Chicken and press Start/Pause. Be sure to shake the

baskets in the middle of cooking.     Remove the wings and place them on a serving plate.     Squeeze fresh lemon juice over the wings and serve.
**Nutrition Info:**Calories: 240 Fat: 15g Carbohydrate: 5g Protein: 19g Sugars: 4g Cholesterol: 60mg

### Italian Chicken

Servings: 4     Cooking Time: 16 Minutes
**Ingredients:**
- 5 chicken thighs
- 1 tbsp. olive oil
- 1/4 cup parmesan; grated
- 1/2 cup sun dried tomatoes
- 2 garlic cloves; minced
- 1 tbsp. thyme; chopped.
- 1/2 cup heavy cream
- 3/4 cup chicken stock
- 1 tsp. red pepper flakes; crushed
- 2 tbsp. basil; chopped
- Salt and black pepper to the taste

**Directions:**
Season chicken with salt and pepper, rub with half of the oil, place in your preheated air fryer at 350 °F and cook for 4 minutes.     Meanwhile; heat up a pan with the rest of the oil over medium high heat, add thyme garlic, pepper flakes, sun dried tomatoes, heavy cream, stock, parmesan, salt and pepper; stir, bring to a simmer, take off heat and transfer to a dish that fits your air fryer. Add chicken thighs on top, introduce in your air fryer and cook at 320 °F, for 12 minutes. Divide among plates and serve with basil sprinkled on top.
**Nutrition Info:**Calories: 272; Fat: 9; Fiber: 12; Carbs: 37; Protein: 23

### Coconut Chicken

Servings: 6     Cooking Time: 4 Hours
**Ingredients:**
- 2 garlic cloves, minced
- Fresh cilantro, minced
- 1/2 cup light coconut milk
- 6 tablespoons sweetened coconut, shredded and toasted
- 2 tablespoons brown sugar
- 6 (about 1-1/2 pounds) boneless skinless chicken thighs
- 2 tablespoons reduced-sodium soy sauce
- 1/8 teaspoon ground cloves

**Directions:**
Mix brown sugar, 1/2 cup light coconut milk, 2 tablespoons soy sauce, 1/8 teaspoon ground cloves and 2 minced cloves of garlic in a bowl.     Add 6 chicken boneless thighs into a Crockpot.     Now pour the mixture of coconut milk over chicken thighs. Cover the cooker and cook for about 4-5 hours on low.     Serve coconut chicken with cilantro and coconut; enjoy!
**Nutrition Info:**201 calories; 10 g fat; 6 g total carbs; 21 g protein

### Spicy Lime Chicken

Servings: 6     Cooking Time: 3 Hours

**Ingredients:**
- 3 tablespoons lime juice
- Fresh cilantro leaves
- 1-1/2 pounds (about 4) boneless skinless chicken breast halves
- 1 teaspoon lime zest, grated
- 2 cups chicken broth
- 1 tablespoon chili powder

**Directions:**
Add chicken breast halves into a slow cooker. Add 1 tablespoon chili powder, 3 tablespoons lime juice and 2 cups chicken broth in a small bowl; mix well and pour over chicken. Cover the cooker and cook for about 3 hours on low. Once done, take chicken out from the cooker and let it cool. Once cooled, shred chicken by using forks and transfer back to the Crockpot. Stir in 1 teaspoon grated lime zest. Serve spicy lime chicken with cilantro and enjoy!

**Nutrition Info:** 132 calories; 3 g fat; 2 g total carbs; 23 g protein

## Crock-pot Slow Cooker Ranch Chicken

Servings: 4     Cooking Time: 4 Hours

**Ingredients:**
- 1 cup chive and onion cream cheese spread
- ½ teaspoon freshly ground black pepper
- 4 boneless chicken breasts
- 1 1-oz package ranch dressing and seasoning mix
- ½ cup low sodium chicken stock

**Directions:**
Spray the Crock-Pot slow cooker with cooking spray and preheat it. Dry chicken with paper towel and transfer it to the Crock-Pot slow cooker. Cook each side, until chicken is browned, for about 4-5 minutes. Add ½ cup low sodium chicken stock, 1 1-oz. package ranch dressing and seasoning mix, 1 cup chive and onion cream cheese spread and ½ teaspoon freshly ground black pepper. Cover the Crock-Pot slow cooker and cook for about 4 hours on Low or until the internal temperature reaches 165 F. Once cooked, take it out from the Crock-Pot slow cooker. Whisk the sauce present in the Crock-Pot slow cooker until smooth. If you need thick sauce, then cook for about 5-10 minutes, with frequent stirring. Garnish chicken with sliced onions and bacon and serve.

**Nutrition Info:** 362 calories; 18.5 g fat; 9.7 g total carbs; 37.3 g protein

## Mustard Chicken With Basil

Servings: 4     Cooking Time: 30 Minutes

**Ingredients:**
- 1 tsp Chicken stock
- 2 Chicken breasts; skinless and boneless chicken breasts: halved
- 1 tbsp Chopped basil
- What you'll need from the store cupboard:
- Salt and black pepper
- 1 tbsp Olive oil
- ½ tsp Garlic powder
- ½ tsp Onion powder
- 1 tsp Dijon mustard

**Directions:**
Press 'Sauté' on the instant pot and add the oil. When it is hot, brown the chicken in it for 2-3 minutes. Mix in the remaining ingredients and seal the lid to cook for 12 minutes at high pressure. Natural release the pressure for 10 minutes, share into plates and serve.

**Nutrition Info:** Calories 34, fat 3.6, carbs 0.7, protein 0.3, fiber 0.1

## Chicken Chili

Servings: 6     Cooking Time: 40 Minutes

**Ingredients:**
- 4 cups low-sodium chicken broth, divided
- 3 cups boiled black beans, divided
- 1 tablespoon extra-virgin olive oil
- 1 large onion, chopped
- 1 jalapeño pepper, seeded and chopped
- 4 garlic cloves, minced
- 1 teaspoon dried thyme, crushed
- 1½ tablespoons ground coriander
- 1 tablespoon ground cumin
- ½ tablespoon red chili powder
- 4 cups cooked chicken, shredded
- 1 tablespoon fresh lime juice
- ¼ cup fresh cilantro, chopped

**Directions:**
In a food processor, add 1 cup of broth and 1 can of black beans and pulse until smooth. Transfer the beans puree into a bowl and set aside. In a large pan, heat the oil over medium heat and sauté the onion and jalapeño for about 4-5 minutes. Add the garlic, spices and sea salt and sauté for about 1 minute. Add the beans puree and remaining broth and bring to a boil. Now, reduce the heat to low and simmer for about 20 minutes. Stir in the remaining can of beans, chicken and lime juice and bring to a boil. Now, reduce the heat to low and simmer for about 5-10 minutes. Serve hot with the garnishing of cilantro. Meal Prep Tip: Transfer the chili into a large bowl and set aside to cool. Divide the chili into 6 containers evenly. Cover the containers and refrigerate for 1-2 days. Reheat in the microwave before serving.

**Nutrition Info:** Calories 356 Total Fat 7.1 g Saturated Fat 1.2 g Cholesterol 72 mg Total Carbs 33 g Sugar 2.7 g Fiber 11.6 g Sodium 130 mg Potassium 662 mg Protein 39.6 g

## Chicken With Cashew Nuts

Servings: 4     Cooking Time: 30 Minutes

**Ingredients:**
- 1 lb chicken cubes
- 2 tbsp soy sauce
- 1 tbsp corn flour
- 2 ½ onion cubes
- 1 carrot, chopped
- ⅓ cup cashew nuts, fried
- 1 capsicum, cut
- 2 tbsp garlic, crushed
- Salt and white pepper

**Directions:**

Marinate the chicken cubes with ½ tbsp of white pepper, ½ tsp salt, 2 tbsp soya sauce, and add 1 tbsp corn flour. Set aside for 25 minutes. Preheat the Air Fryer to 380 F and transfer the marinated chicken. Add the garlic, the onion, the capsicum, and the carrot; fry for 5-6 minutes. Roll it in the cashew nuts before serving.

**Nutrition Info:** Calories: 425; Carbs: 25g; Fat: 35g; Protein: 53g

## Chuck And Veggies

Servings: 2     Cooking Time: 9 Hours

**Ingredients:**
- ¼ cup dry red wine
- ¼ teaspoon salt
- 8 oz. boneless lean chuck roast
- ¼ teaspoon black pepper
- 8 oz. frozen pepper stir-fry
- 1 teaspoon Worcestershire sauce
- 8 oz. whole mushrooms
- 1 teaspoon instant coffee granules
- 1 1/4 cups fresh green beans, trimmed
- 1 dried bay leaf

**Directions:**
Mix all the ingredients except salt in a bowl; combine well and then transfer to a slow cooker.     Cover the cooker and cook for about 9 hours on low and 4 1/2 hours on high, until beef is completely cooked through and tender.     Stir in ¼ teaspoon salt gently. Take out the vegetables and beef and transfer to 2 shallow bowls. Pour liquid into the skillet; boil it lightly and cook until liquid reduces to ¼ cup, for about 1 1/2 minutes.     Pour over veggies and beef. Discard bay leaf and serve.

**Nutrition Info:** 215 calories; 5 g fat; 17 g total carbs; 26 g protein

## Chicken & Broccoli Bake

Servings: 6     Cooking Time: 45 Minutes

**Ingredients:**
- 6 (6-ounce) boneless, skinless chicken breasts
- 3 broccoli heads, cut into florets
- 4 garlic cloves, minced
- ¼ cup olive oil
- 1 teaspoon dried oregano, crushed
- 1 teaspoon dried rosemary, crushed
- Sea Salt and ground black pepper, as required

**Directions:**
Preheat the oven to 375 degrees F. Grease a large baking dish.     In a large bowl, add all the ingredients and toss to coat well.     In the bottom of prepared baking dish, arrange the broccoli florets and top with chicken breasts in a single layer.     Bake for about 45 minutes. Remove from the oven and set aside for about 5 minutes before serving.     Meal Prep Tip: Remove the baking dish from the oven and set aside to cool completely. In 6 containers, divide the chicken breasts and broccoli evenly and refrigerate for about 2 days. Reheat in microwave before serving.

**Nutrition Info:** Calories 443 Total Fat 21.5 g Saturated Fat 4.7 g Cholesterol 151 mg Total Carbs 9.4 g Sugar 2.2g Fiber 3.6 g Sodium 189 mg Potassium 831 mg Protein 53 g

## Rosemary Lemon Chicken

Servings: 4     Cooking Time: 14 Minutes

**Ingredients:**
- 1 kg chicken breast halves
- 1 lemon, peeled and sliced into rounds
- 1/2 orange, peeled and sliced into rounds, or to taste
- 3 cloves roasted garlic, or to taste
- salt and ground black pepper to taste
- 1 1/2 tablespoons olive oil, or to taste
- 1 1/2 teaspoons agave syrup, or to taste (optional)
- 1/4 cup water
- 2 sprigs fresh rosemary, stemmed, or to taste

**Directions:**
Place chicken in the Instant Pot. Add lemon, orange, and garlic; season with salt and pepper. Drizzle olive oil and agave syrup (if using) on top. Add water and rosemary. Put the lid on the cooker and Lock in place.     Select the "Meat" and "Stew" settings for High pressure, and cook for 14 minutes. Allow pressure to release naturally, about 20 minutes.

**Nutrition Info:** Calories 325 Fat 5 g Carbohydrates 20 g Sugar 2 g Protein 10 g Cholesterol 33 mg

## Ginger Flavored Chicken

Servings: 6     Cooking Time: 15 Minutes

**Ingredients:**
- 1 kg boneless, skinless chicken breasts (frozen OR thawed)
- 6 tablespoons soy sauce
- 3 tablespoons rice vinegar
- 1/2 tablespoon honey
- 3 tablespoons water, broth, or orange juice
- 2 tablespoons chopped fresh ginger
- 6 cloves garlic, minced
- 3 teaspoons corn starch

**Directions:**
Place chicken breasts in Instant Pot.     In a small mixing bowl, whisk together: vinegar, soy sauce, honey, water, ginger and garlic. Pour mixture over chicken and coat evenly.     Secure lid on Instant Pot and cook at High pressure for 15 minutes. When the meat is cooked, release steam.     Remove chicken breasts and place on a cutting board. Bring remaining sauce in pan up to a simmer (use the Saute feature on an electric cooker). Combine cornstarch with 3 teaspoons cold water and then pour mixture into pan. Simmer until sauce is thickened and the turn off heat.     Shred chicken and return to pot with sauce.

**Nutrition Info:** Calories 313 Fat 25.6 g Carbohydrates 15.6 g Sugar 7 g Protein 8 g Cholesterol 36 mg

## Crock-pot Slow Cooker Tex-mex Chicken

Servings: 6     Cooking Time: 4 Hours 40 Minutes

**Ingredients:**
- 4 tablespoons cup water
- 1 teaspoon ground cumin
- 1 lb boneless chicken thighs, visible fat removed, rinsed, and patted dry
- 1 (10 oz) can diced tomatoes and green chilies

- 1 (16 oz) package frozen onion and pepper strips, thawed

**Directions:**
Spray a skillet with cooking spray and turn heat flame on. Place chicken thighs into the skillet and cook each side until browned over medium heat. Once browned, take out from the skillet. To the same skillet, add peppers and onions and cook until tender. Transfer cooked peppers and onions into 4- to 5-quart Crock-Pot slow cooker followed by chicken thighs on top. Place tomatoes along with 4 tablespoons of water over chicken. Cook for about 4 hours on Low. Add 1 teaspoon ground cumin and cook further for half an hour. Once done, take it out and serve right away!

**Nutrition Info:**121 calories; 3.2 g fat; 6.4 g total carbs; 16 g protein

## Slow-cooker Chicken Fajita Burritos

Servings: 8     Cooking Time: 6 Hrs

**Ingredients:**
- 1 teaspoon cumin
- 1 cup cheddar cheese + 2 tablespoons reduced-fat, shredded
- 1 lb. chicken strips, skinless and boneless
- 8 large low-carb tortillas
- 1 green pepper, sliced
- 1 can (15 oz) black beans, rinsed and drained
- 1 red pepper, sliced
- 1/3 cup water
- 1 medium onion, sliced
- ½ cup salsa
- 1 tablespoon chili powder
- 1 teaspoon garlic powder

**Directions:**
Place strips of chicken breast in a slow-cooker. Top chicken with all ingredients mentioned above except for cheese and tortillas. Cover the cooker and cook for approximately 6 hours, until done. Shred chicken with a fork. Serve half cup of chicken on each tortilla along with the bean mixture. Finish with 2 tablespoons of shredded cheese, then fold tortilla into a burrito.

**Nutrition Info:**250 calories; 7 g fat; 31 g total carbs; 28 g protein

## Chicken With Chickpeas

Servings: 4     Cooking Time: 36 Minutes

**Ingredients:**
- 2 tablespoons olive oil
- 1 pound skinless, boneless chicken breast, cubed
- 2 carrots, peeled and sliced
- 1 onion, chopped
- 2 celery stalks, chopped
- 2 garlic cloves, chopped
- 1 tablespoon fresh ginger root, minced
- ½ teaspoon dried oregano, crushed
- ¾ teaspoon ground cumin
- ½ teaspoon paprika
- ¼-13 teaspoon cayenne pepper
- ¼ teaspoon ground turmeric
- 1 cup tomatoes, crushed

- 1½ cups low-sodium chicken broth
- 1 zucchini, sliced
- 1 cup boiled chickpeas, drained
- 1 tablespoon fresh lemon juice

**Directions:**
In a large nonstick pan, heat the oil over medium heat and cook the chicken cubes for about 4-5 minutes. With a slotted spoon, transfer the chicken cubes onto a plate. In the same pan, add the carrot, onion, celery and garlic and sauté for about 4-5 minutes. Add the ginger, oregano and spices and sauté for about 1 minute. Add the chicken, tomato and broth and bring to a boil. Now, reduce the heat to low and simmer for about 10 minutes. Add the zucchini and chickpeas and simmer, covered for about 15 minutes. Stir in the lemon juice and serve hot. Meal Prep Tip: Transfer the chicken mixture into a large bowl and set aside to cool. Divide the mixture into 4 containers evenly. Cover the containers and refrigerate for 1-2 days. Reheat in the microwave before serving.

**Nutrition Info:**Calories 308 Total Fat 12.3 g Saturated Fat 2.7 g Cholesterol 66 mg Total Carbs 19 g Sugar 5.3g Fiber 4.7 g Sodium 202 mg Potassium 331 mg Protein 30.7 g

## Garlic Soy-glazed Chicken

Servings: 6     Cooking Time: 25 Minutes

**Ingredients:**
- 2 pounds' boneless chicken thighs
- What you'll need from the store cupboard:
- Salt and pepper
- 1 tablespoon minced garlic
- ¼ cup soy sauce
- ¾ cup apple cider vinegar

**Directions:**
Season the chicken with salt and pepper, then add it to the Instant Pot, skin-side down. Whisk together the apple cider vinegar, soy sauce, and garlic then add to the pot. Close and lock the lid, then press the Manual button and adjust the timer to 15 minutes. When the timer goes off, let the pressure vent naturally. When the pot has depressurized, open the lid. Remove the chicken to a baking sheet and place under the broiler for 3 to 5 minutes until the skin is crisp. Meanwhile, turn the Instant Pot on to Sauté and cook until the sauce thickens, stirring as needed. Serve the chicken with the sauce spooned over it.

**Nutrition Info:**calories 335 fat 23g protein 27.5g carbs 1.5g fiber 0g net carbs 1.5g

## Chicken Tikka Masala

Servings: 4     Cooking Time: 10 Minutes

**Ingredients:**
- 2 tablespoons olive oil
- 1 small onion, diced
- 3 cloves garlic, minced
- 1 (2-inch) piece fresh ginger, peeled and grated
- 1/2 cup chicken broth,
- 1 1/2 tablespoons garam masala
- 1 teaspoon paprika
- 1/2 teaspoon ground turmeric

- 1/2 teaspoon salt
- 1/4 teaspoon cayenne pepper
- 750 gr boneless, skinless chicken meat, cut into small pieces
- 450 g can tomatoes, juices included
- 1/2 cup coconut milk
- Fresh cilantro, chopped

**Directions:**
Set the cooker to the Sauté. Add the oil, and when it's hot, add the onion and sauté until softened, about 3 minutes. Add the garlic and ginger and cook until soft. Add half of the chicken broth. Cook for couple of minutes, stirring all the time, add the garam masala, paprika, turmeric, salt, and cayenne pepper, and stir to combine. Add the chicken and the remaining chicken broth and the tomatoes. Close and lock the lid. Pressure-cook for 10 minutes at High pressure. When it's cooked, do a quick release of the pressure. Stir the coconut milk into the sauce. Serving suggestion: Serve on a bed of cauliflower "rice", or boiled potatoes.
**Nutrition Info:**Calories 245 Fat 25 g Carbohydrates 12.6 g Sugar 4 g Protein 5 g Cholesterol 35 mg

## Lemon Garlic Turkey

Servings: 4    Cooking Time: 5 Minutes
**Ingredients:**
- 4 turkey breasts fillet
- 2 cloves garlic, minced
- 1 tablespoon olive oil
- 3 tablespoons lemon juice
- 1 oz. Parmesan cheese, shredded
- Pepper to taste
- 1 tablespoon fresh sage, snipped
- 1 teaspoon lemon zest

**Directions:**
Pound the turkey breast until flat. In a bowl, mix the olive oil, garlic and lemon juice. Add the turkey to the bowl. Marinate for 1 hour. Broil for 5 minutes until turkey is fully cooked. Sprinkle cheese on top on the last minute of cooking. In a bowl, mix the pepper, sage and lemon zest. Sprinkle this mixture on top of the turkey before serving.
**Nutrition Info:**Calories 188 Total Fat 7 g Saturated Fat 2 g Cholesterol 71 mg Sodium 173 mg Total Carbohydrate 2 g Dietary Fiber 0 g Total Sugars 0 g Protein 29 g Potassium 264 mg

## Whole Roasted Chicken

Servings: 6    Cooking Time: 10 Minutes
**Ingredients:**
- 1 whole chicken (about 2 kg)
- 1 tablespoon chopped fresh rosemary
- 1 1/2-2 tablespoons olive oil, plus a bit more for drizzling in pan
- 4-6 cloves garlic
- 1/2 teaspoon paprika
- Salt and pepper to taste
- Zest from 1 lemon
- 1 cup chicken broth
- 1 large onion, quartered

**Directions:**

Rinse the chicken with cold water and pat dry with paper towels. Place in baking pan and set aside. Preheat Instant Pot and go to Saute mode. In a small bowl combine rosemary, olive oil, garlic, paprika, salt, pepper, and lemon zest. After removing the zest, cut lemon in half and stuff in cavity of chicken. Spread spice mixture all over the chicken, spreading evenly. Drizzle some olive oil in your hot pan and place chicken breast-side down into pot. Leave for 3-4 minutes, until golden brown. Flip chicken over and bake the other side. Remove chicken from pan and set onto the baking dish where it was before. Add broth to pan. Place onion on bottom of pan, place chicken on top (breast-side up) and secure lid. Cook on High pressure for 6 minutes per pound. When it's cooked, wait for 10 minutes before releasing steam. Remove chicken and wait for at least 5 minutes before slicing.
**Nutrition Info:**Calories 301 Fat 27.2 g Carbohydrates 13.6 g Sugar 6 g Protein 4.9 g Cholesterol 33 mg

## Fried Chicken Tamari And Mustard

Servings: 4    Cooking Time: 1h 20 Minutes
**Ingredients:**
- 1kg of very small chopped chicken
- Tamari Sauce
- Original mustard
- Ground pepper
- 1 lemon
- Flour
- Extra virgin olive oil

**Directions:**
Put the chicken in a bowl, you can put the chicken with or without the skin, to everyone's taste. Add a generous stream of tamari, one or two tablespoons of mustard, a little ground pepper and a splash of lemon juice. Link everything very well and let macerate an hour. Pass the chicken pieces for flour and place in the air fryer basket. Put 20 minutes at 200 degrees. At half time, move the chicken from the basket. Do not crush the chicken, it is preferable to make two or three batches of chicken to pile up and do not fry the pieces well.
**Nutrition Info:**Calories: 100 Fat: 6g Carbohydrates 0g Protein: 18g Sugar: 0g

## Herbed Chicken

Servings: 4    Cooking Time: 50 Minutes
**Ingredients:**
- 1 whole chicken
- 1 tsp. garlic powder
- 1 tsp. onion powder
- 1/2 tsp. thyme; dried
- 1 tsp. rosemary; dried
- 1 tbsp. lemon juice
- 2 tbsp. olive oil
- Salt and black pepper to the taste

**Directions:**
Season chicken with salt and pepper, rub with thyme, rosemary, garlic powder and onion powder, rub with lemon juice and olive oil and leave aside for 30 minutes. Put chicken in your air fryer and cook at 360 °F, for 20

minutes on each side. Leave chicken aside to cool down, carve and serve.

**Nutrition Info:**Calories: 390; Fat: 10; Fiber: 5; Carbs: 22; Protein: 20

## Juicy Whole Chicken

Servings: 6     Cooking Time: 30 Minutes
**Ingredients:**
- 2 tbsp olive oil
- 300 ml chicken broth
- 3 red potatoes
- 1 chicken, whole
- Spices of your choice, eg thyme, oregano, salt, garlic salt

**Directions:**
Put your Instant Pot on Saute, Low Setting.     Add olive oil and when it's hot, add chicken to the pot and lightly cook for about 2 minutes. Repeat with the other side. Turn off by pressing Cancel.     Remove browned meat from Instant Pot and add chicken broth, potatoes, and the chicken (whole or in pieces). Chicken should be on top of the potatoes.     Close lid, make sure steam valve is secure, and set to Poultry, normal setting, for 25 minutes. When it's cooked, do a quick release

**Nutrition Info:**Calories 301 Fat 27.2 g Carbohydrates 13.6 g Sugar 6 g Protein 4.9 g Cholesterol 33 mg

## Tasty Chicken Tenders

Servings: 4     Cooking Time: 25 Minutes.
**Ingredients:**
- 1 ½ lbs chicken tenders
- 1 tbsp. extra virgin olive oil
- 1 tsp. rotisserie chicken seasoning
- 2 tbsp. BBQ sauce

**Directions:**
Add all ingredients except oil in a zip-lock bag.     Seal bag and place in the refrigerator for 2-3 hours.     Heat oil in a large pan over medium heat.     Cook marinated chicken tenders in a pan until lightly brown and cooked.

**Nutrition Info:**Calories 365 Fat 16.1 g, Carbohydrates 2.8 g, Sugar 2 g, Protein 49.2 g, Cholesterol 151 mg

## Salted Biscuit Pie Turkey Chops

Servings: 4     Cooking Time: 20 Minutes
**Ingredients:**
- 8 large turkey chops
- 300 gr of crackers
- 2 eggs
- Extra virgin olive oil
- Salt
- Ground pepper

**Directions:**
Put the turkey chops on the worktable, and salt and pepper.     Beat the eggs in a bowl.     Crush the cookies in the Thermo mix with a few turbo strokes until they are made grit, or you can crush them with the blender. Put the cookies in a bowl.     Pass the chops through the beaten egg and then passed them through the crushed cookies. Press well so that the empanada is perfect. Paint the empanada with a silicone brush and extra

virgin olive oil.     Put the chops in the basket of the air fryer, not all will enter. They will be done in batches. Select 200 degrees, 15 minutes.     When you have all the chops made, serve.

**Nutrition Info:**Calories: 126 Fat: 6g Carbohydrates 0g Protein: 18g Sugar: 0g

## Creamy Chicken, Peas And Rice

Servings: 4     Cooking Time: 20 Minutes
**Ingredients:**
- 1 lb. chicken breasts; skinless, boneless and cut into quarters
- 1 cup white rice; already cooked
- 1 cup chicken stock
- 1/4 cup parsley; chopped.
- 2 cups peas; frozen
- 1 ½ cups parmesan; grated
- 1 tbsp. olive oil
- 3 garlic cloves; minced
- 1 yellow onion; chopped
- 1/2 cup white wine
- 1/4 cup heavy cream
- Salt and black pepper to the taste

**Directions:**
Season chicken breasts with salt and pepper, drizzle half of the oil over them, rub well, put in your air fryer's basket and cook them at 360 °F, for 6 minutes.     Heat up a pan with the rest of the oil over medium high heat, add garlic, onion, wine, stock, salt, pepper and heavy cream; stir, bring to a simmer and cook for 9 minutes.     Transfer chicken breasts to a heat proof dish that fits your air fryer, add peas, rice and cream mix over them, toss, sprinkle parmesan and parsley all over, place in your air fryer and cook at 420 °F, for 10 minutes. Divide among plates and serve hot.

**Nutrition Info:**Calories: 313; Fat: 12; Fiber: 14; Carbs: 27; Protein: 44

## Oregano Flavored Chicken Olives

Servings: 4     Cooking Time: 15 Minutes
**Ingredients:**
- 2 pieces (without skin and bones) Chicken breasts
- 2 pieces Eggplants
- 1 tbsp Oregano
- 1 cup Tomato passata
- What you'll need from the store cupboard:
- Salt and Black pepper to taste
- 2 tbsp Olive oil

**Directions:**
In the instant pot mix all the ingredients, then cover them and cook for 20 minutes on high temperature. Release the pressure gradually for 10 minutes then split them among your plates before eating.

**Nutrition Info:**Calories: 362, Fat: 16.1, Fiber: 4.4g, Carbs: 5.4g, Protein: 36.4g

## Chinese Stuffed Chicken

Servings: 8     Cooking Time: 30 Minutes
**Ingredients:**
- 1 whole chicken

- 10 wolfberries
- 2 red chilies; chopped
- 4 ginger slices
- 1 yam; cubed
- 1 tsp. soy sauce
- 3 tsp. sesame oil
- Salt and white pepper to the taste

**Directions:**
Season chicken with salt, pepper, rub with soy sauce and sesame oil and stuff with wolfberries, yam cubes, chilies and ginger.    Place in your air fryer, cook at 400 °F, for 20 minutes and then at 360 °F, for 15 minutes. Carve chicken, divide among plates and serve.
**Nutrition Info:**Calories: 320; Fat: 12; Fiber: 17; Carbs: 22; Protein: 12

## Chicken & Spinach

Servings: 4    Cooking Time: 13 Minutes
**Ingredients:**
- 2 tablespoons olive oil
- 1 lb. chicken breast fillet, sliced into small pieces
- Salt and pepper to taste
- 4 cloves garlic, minced
- 1 tablespoon lemon juice
- ½ cup dry white wine
- 1 teaspoon lemon zest
- 10 cups fresh spinach, chopped
- 4 tablespoons Parmesan cheese, grated

**Directions:**
Pour oil in a pan over medium heat.    Season chicken with salt and pepper.    Cook in the pan for 7 minutes until golden on both sides.    Add the garlic and cook for 1 minute.    Stir in the lemon juice and wine.    Sprinkle lemon zest on top.    Simmer for 5 minutes.    Add the spinach and cook until wilted.    Serve with Parmesan cheese.
**Nutrition Info:**Calories 334 Total Fat 12 g Saturated Fat 3 g Cholesterol 67 mg Sodium 499 mg Total Carbohydrate 25 g Dietary Fiber 2 g Total Sugars 1 g Protein 29 g Potassium 685 mg

## Air Fried Chicken With Honey And Lemon

Servings: 4    Cooking Time: 50 Minutes
**Ingredients:**
- The Stuffing:
- 1 whole chicken, 3 lb
- 2 red and peeled onions
- 2 tbsp olive oil
- 2 apricots
- 1 zucchini
- 1 apple
- 2 cloves finely chopped garlic
- Fresh chopped thyme
- Salt and pepper
- The Marinade:
- 5 oz honey
- juice from 1 lemon
- 2 tbsp olive oil
- Salt and pepper

**Directions:**

For the stuffing, chop all ingredients into tiny pieces. Transfer to a large bowl and add the olive oil. Season with salt and black pepper. Fill the cavity of the chicken with the stuffing, without packing it tightly.    Place the chicken in the Air Fryer and cook for 35 minutes at 340 F. Warm the honey and the lemon juice in a large pan; season with salt and pepper. Reduce the temperature of the Air Fryer to 320 F.    Brush the chicken with some of the honey-lemon marinade and return it to the fryer. Cook for another 70 minutes; brush the chicken every 20-25 minutes with the marinade. Garnish with parsley, and serve with potatoes.
**Nutrition Info:**Calories: 342; Carbs: 68g; Fat: 28g; Protein: 33g

## Honey Mustard Chicken

Servings: 4    Cooking Time: 12 Minutes
**Ingredients:**
- 2 tablespoons honey mustard
- 2 teaspoons olive oil
- Salt to taste
- 1 lb. chicken tenders
- 1 lb. baby carrots, steamed
- Chopped parsley

**Directions:**
Preheat your oven to 450 degrees F.    Mix honey mustard, olive oil and salt.    Coat the chicken tenders with the mixture.    Place the chicken on a single layer on the baking pan.    Bake for 10 to 12 minutes.    Serve with steamed carrots and garnish with parsley.
**Nutrition Info:**Calories 366 Total Fat 8 g Saturated Fat 2 g Cholesterol 63 mg Sodium 543 mg Total Carbohydrate 46 g Dietary Fiber 8 g Total Sugars 13 g Protein 33 g Potassium 377 mg

## Greek Chicken Lettuce Wraps

Servings: 4    Cooking Time: 8 Minutes
**Ingredients:**
- 2 tablespoons freshly squeezed lemon juice
- 1 teaspoon lemon zest
- 5 teaspoons olive oil, divided
- 3 teaspoons garlic, minced and divided
- 1 teaspoon dried oregano
- ¼ teaspoon red pepper, crushed
- 1 lb. chicken tenders
- 1 cucumber, sliced in half and grated
- Salt and pepper to taste
- ¾ cup non-fat Greek yogurt
- 2 teaspoons fresh mint, chopped
- 2 teaspoons fresh dill, chopped
- 4 lettuce leaves
- ½ cup red onion, sliced
- 1 cup tomatoes, chopped

**Directions:**
In a bowl, mix the lemon juice, lemon zest, half of oil, half of garlic, and red pepper.    Coat the chicken with the marinade.    Marinate it for 1 hour.    Toss grated cucumber in salt.    Squeeze to release liquid.    Add the yogurt, dill, salt, pepper, remaining garlic and remaining oil.    Grill the chicken for 4 minutes per side. Shred the chicken and put on top of the lettuce leaves.

Top with the yogurt mixture, onion and tomatoes. Wrap the lettuce leaves and secure with a toothpick.
**Nutrition Info:**Calories 353 Total Fat 9 g Saturated Fat 1 g Cholesterol 58 mg Sodium 559 mg Total Carbohydrate 33 g Dietary Fiber 6 g Total Sugars 6 g Protein 37 g Potassium 459 mg

## Spicy Honey Orange Chicken

Servings: 4    Cooking Time: 10 Minutes
**Ingredients:**
- 1 ½ pounds chicken breast, washed and sliced
- Parsley to taste
- 1 cup coconut, shredded
- ¾ cup breadcrumbs
- 2 whole eggs, beaten
- ½ cup flour
- ½ tsp pepper
- Salt to taste
- ½ cup orange marmalade
- 1 tbsp red pepper flakes
- ¼ cup honey
- 3 tbsp dijon mustard

**Directions:**
Preheat your Air Fryer to 400 F. In a mixing bowl, combine coconut, flour, salt, parsley and pepper. In another bowl, add the beaten eggs. Place breadcrumbs in a third bowl. Dredge chicken in egg mix, flour and finally in the breadcrumbs. Place the chicken in the Air Fryer cooking basket and bake for 15 minutes.    In a separate bowl, mix honey, orange marmalade, mustard and pepper flakes. Cover chicken with marmalade mixture and fry for 5 more minutes. Enjoy!
**Nutrition Info:**Calories: 246; Carbs: 21g; Fat: 6g; Protein: 25g

## Chicken Soup

Servings: 6    Cooking Time: 30 Minutes
**Ingredients:**
- 4 lbs Chicken, cut into pieces
- 5 carrots, sliced thick
- 8 cups of water
- 2 celery stalks, sliced 1 inch thick
- 2 large onions, sliced

**Directions:**
In a large pot add chicken, water, and salt. Bring to boil. Add celery and onion in the pot and stir well.    Turn heat to medium-low and simmer for 30 minutes.    Add carrots and cover pot with a lid and simmer for 40 minutes.    Remove Chicken from the pot and remove bones and cut Chicken into bite-size pieces.    Return chicken into the pot and stir well.    Serve and enjoy.
**Nutrition Info:**Calories: 89 Fat: 6.33g Carbohydrates: 0g Protein: 7.56g Sugar: 0g    Cholesterol: 0mg

## Ginger Chili Broccoli

Servings: 5    Cooking Time: 15 Minutes
**Ingredients:**
- 8 cups broccoli florets
- 1/2 cup olive oil
- 2 fresh lime juice
- 2 tbsp fresh ginger, grated
- 2 tsp chili pepper, chopped

**Directions:**
Add broccoli florets into the steamer and steam for 8 minutes.    Meanwhile, for dressing in a small bowl, combine limejuice, oil, ginger, and chili pepper.    Add steamed broccoli in a large bowl then pour dressing over broccoli. Toss well.
**Nutrition Info:**Calories 239 Fat 20.8 g Carbohydrates 13.7 g Sugar 3 g Protein 4.5 g Cholesterol 0 mg

## Italian Style Chicken Breast

Servings: 3    Cooking Time: 15 Minutes
**Ingredients:**
- 1 tablespoon olive oil
- 3 boneless, skinless chicken breasts
- 1/4 teaspoon garlic powder and regular salt per breast
- dash black pepper
- 1/8 teaspoon dried oregano
- 1/8 teaspoon dried basil
- 250 ml water

**Directions:**
Set the Instant Pot to Saute, and add oil to the pot. Season one side of the chicken breasts and once the oil is hot, carefully add the chicken breasts, seasoned side down, to the pot.    In the meantime, season the second side.    Cook about 3 to 4 minutes on each side, and remove from pot with the tongs.    Add 250 ml water to the pot, plus the trivet.    Place the chicken on the trivet. Lock the lid, and cook on manual High for 5 minutes. Allow the chicken to naturally release for a few minutes, and then quick release the rest.    Remove from the pot and wait for at least 5 minutes before slicing.
**Nutrition Info:**Calories 202 Fat 29 g Carbohydrates 13.6 g Sugar 6 g Protein 4.9 g Cholesterol 33 mg

## Garlic Chives Chicken

Servings: 4    Cooking Time: 10 Minutes
**Ingredients:**
- 1 lb. (no skin and bones) Chicken breast
- 1 tbsp Chives
- 1 cup Chicken stock
- 1 cup Coconut cream
- 3 tbsp Garlic cloves (sliced)
- What you'll need from the store cupboard:
- 1 and a half tbsp Balsamic vinegar
- Salt and Black pepper to taste

**Directions:**
In the instant pot, mix the chicken with all the remaining ingredients, then cover them and cook for 20 minutes on high temperature.    Release the pressure gradually for 10 minutes then split them among your plates before eating.
**Nutrition Info:**Calories: 360, Fat: 22.1, Fiber: 1.4g, Carbs: 4.1g, Protein: 34.5g

## Breaded Chicken Fillets

Servings: 4    Cooking Time: 25 Minutes
**Ingredients:**

- 3 small chicken breasts or 2 large chicken breasts
- Salt
- Ground pepper
- 3 garlic cloves
- 1 lemon
- Beaten eggs
- Breadcrumbs
- Extra virgin olive oil

**Directions:**
Cut the breasts into fillets. Put in a bowl and add the lemon juice, chopped garlic cloves and pepper. Flirt well and leave 10 minutes. Beat the eggs and put breadcrumbs on another plate. Pass the chicken breast fillets through the beaten egg and the breadcrumbs. When you have them all breaded, start to fry. Paint the breaded breasts with a silicone brush and extra virgin olive oil. Place a batch of fillets in the basket of the air fryer and select 10 minutes 180 degrees. Turn around and leave another 5 minutes at 180 degrees.
**Nutrition Info:**Calories: 120 Fat: 6g Carbohydrates 0g Protein: 18g Sugar: 0g

## Chicken Wings With Garlic Parmesan

Servings: 3      Cooking Time: 25 Minutes
**Ingredients:**
- 25g cornstarch
- 20g grated Parmesan cheese
- 9g garlic powder
- Salt and pepper to taste
- 680g chicken wings
- Nonstick Spray Oil

**Directions:**
Select Preheat, set the temperature to 200 °C and press Start / Pause. Combine corn starch, Parmesan, garlic powder, salt, and pepper in a bowl. Mix the chicken wings in the seasoning and dip until well coated. Spray the baskets and the air fryer with oil spray and add the wings, sprinkling the tops of the wings as well. Select Chicken and press Start/Pause. Be sure to shake the baskets in the middle of cooking. Sprinkle with what's left of the Parmesan mix and serve.
**Nutrition Info:**Calories: 204 Fat: 15g Carbohydrates: 1g Proteins: 12g Sugar: 0g Cholesterol: 63mg

## Chicken Salad

Servings: 6      Cooking Time: 30 Minutes
**Ingredients:**
- 1 kg chicken breast
- 125 ml chicken broth
- 1 teaspoon salt
- ½ teaspoon black pepper

**Directions:**
Add all of the ingredients to the Instant Pot. Secure the lid, close the pressure valve and cook for 20 minutes at High pressure. Quick release pressure. Shred the chicken. Store in an air-tight container with the liquid to help keep the meat moist.
**Nutrition Info:**Calories 356 Fat 27.2 g Carbohydrates 13.6 g Sugar 3 g Protein 4.9 g Cholesterol 5 mg

## Duck With Garlic And Onion Sauce

Servings: 4      Cooking Time: 20 Minutes
**Ingredients:**
- 2 tbsp Coriander
- 2 pieces Spring onions
- 1 lb. (no skin and bones) Duck legs
- 2 pieces Garlic cloves
- 2 tbsp Tomato passata
- What you'll need from the store cupboard:
- 2 tbsp Melted ghee

**Directions:**
Put the instant pot on Sauté option, then put the ghee and cook it. After that, put the spring onions and the other ingredients excluding the tomato passata and the meat then heat it for 5 minutes. Put the meat and cook for 5 minutes. Put the sauce then cover it and heat it for 25 minutes on high temperature. Release the pressure gradually for 10 minutes then split them among your plates before eating.
**Nutrition Info:**Calories: 263, Fat: 13.2g, Fiber: 0.2g, Carbs: 1.1g, Protein: 33.5g

## Crock-pot Slow Cooker Mulligatawny Soup

Servings: 8      Cooking Time: 6 Hours
**Ingredients:**
- 2 whole cloves
- 1/4 cup green pepper, chopped
- 1 carton (32 oz.) low-sodium chicken broth
- 1/4 teaspoon pepper
- 1 can (14 1/2 oz.) diced tomatoes
- 1/2 teaspoon sugar
- 2 cups cubed cooked chicken
- 1 teaspoon curry powder
- 1 large tart green apple, peeled and chopped
- 1 teaspoon salt
- 1/4 cup onion, finely chopped
- 2 teaspoon lemon juice
- 1/4 cup carrot, chopped
- 1 tablespoon fresh parsley, minced

**Directions:**
Add all ingredients in a 3- or 4-qt. Crock-Pot slow cooker and combine well. Cover the cooker and cook for about 6-8 hours on Low. Once done, remove cloves and serve.
**Nutrition Info:**107 calories; 2 g fat; 10 g total carbs; 12 g protein

## Lemon Chicken With Basil

Servings: 4      Cooking Time: 1h
**Ingredients:**
- 1kg chopped chicken
- 1 or 2 lemons
- Basil, salt, and ground pepper
- Extra virgin olive oil

**Directions:**
Put the chicken in a bowl with a jet of extra virgin olive oil. Put salt, pepper, and basil. Bind well and let stand for at least 30 minutes stirring occasionally. Put the pieces of chicken in the air fryer basket and take the air fryer Select 30 minutes. Occasionally remove.

Take out and put another batch. Do the same operation.

**Nutrition Info:**Calories: 126 Fat: 6g Carbohydrates 0g Protein: 18g Sugar: 0g

## Chicken, Oats & Chickpeas Meatloaf

Servings: 4    Cooking Time: 1¼ Hours
**Ingredients:**
- ½ cup cooked chickpeas
- 2 egg whites
- 2½ teaspoons poultry seasoning
- Ground black pepper, as required
- 10 ounce lean ground chicken
- 1 cup red bell pepper, seeded and minced
- 1 cup celery stalk, minced
- 1/3 cup steel-cut oats
- 1 cup tomato puree, divided
- 2 tablespoons dried onion flakes, crushed
- 1 tablespoon prepared mustard

**Directions:**
Preheat the oven to 350 degrees F. Grease a 9x5-inch loaf pan.    In a food processor, add chickpeas, egg whites, poultry seasoning and black pepper and pulse until smooth.    Transfer the mixture into a large bowl. Add the chicken, veggies oats, ½ cup of tomato puree and onion flakes and mix until well combined. Transfer the mixture into prepared loaf pan evenly. With your hands, press, down the mixture slightly.    In another bowl mix together mustard and remaining tomato puree.    Place the mustard mixture over loaf pan evenly.    Bake for about 1-1¼ hours or until desired doneness.    Remove from the oven and set aside for about 5 minutes before slicing.g.    Cut into desired sized slices and serve.    Meal Prep Tip: In a resealable plastic bag, place the cooled meatloaf slices and seal the bag. Refrigerate for about 2-4 days. Reheat in the microwave on High for about 1 minute before serving.

**Nutrition Info:**Calories 229 Total Fat 5.6 g Saturated Fat 1.4 g Cholesterol 50 mg Total Carbs 23.7 g Sugar 5.2 g Fiber 4.7 g Sodium 227 mg Potassium 509 mg Protein 21.4 g

## Turkey And Spring Onions Mix

Servings: 4    Cooking Time: 10 Minutes
**Ingredients:**
- Cilantro
- 4 pieces Spring onions (sliced)
- 1 piece (no skin and bones) Turkey breast
- 1 cup Tomato passata
- What you'll need from the store cupboard:
- 2 tbsp Avocado oil
- Salt and Black pepper to taste

**Directions:**
Put the instant pot on Sauté option, then put the oil and cook it. After that, put the meat then heat it for 5 minutes. Put the other ingredients, then cover it and heat it for 20 minutes on high temperature.    Release the pressure gradually for 10 minutes then split them among your plates before eating.

**Nutrition Info:**Calories: 222, Fat: 6.7g, Fiber: 1.6g, Carbs: 4.8g, Protein: 34.4g

## Chinese Chicken Wings

Servings: 6    Cooking Time: 10 Minutes
**Ingredients:**
- 16 chicken wings
- 2 tbsp. honey
- 2 tbsp. soy sauce
- Salt and black pepper to the taste
- 1/4 tsp. white pepper
- 3 tbsp. lime juice

**Directions:**
In a bowl, mix honey with soy sauce, salt, black and white pepper and lime juice, whisk well, add chicken pieces, toss to coat and keep in the fridge for 2 hours. Transfer chicken to your air fryer, cook at 370 °F, for 6 minutes on each side, increase heat to 400 °F and cook for 3 minutes more. Serve hot.

**Nutrition Info:**Calories: 372; Fat: 9; Fiber: 10; Carbs: 37; Protein: 24

## Basil Chili Chicken

Servings: 4    Cooking Time: 20 Minutes
**Ingredients:**
- half cup Chicken stock
- 1 lb. Chicken breast
- 2 tsp Sweet paprika
- 1 cup Coconut cream
- 2 tbsp Basil (sliced)
- What you'll need from the store cupboard:
- Salt and Black pepper to taste
- 1 tbsp Chili powder

**Directions:**
In your instant pot, mix the chicken with the other ingredients, then stir them a little, then cover them then heat for 20 minutes on high temperature.    Release the pressure gradually for 10 minutes then split them among plates before you eat them.

**Nutrition Info:**Calories: 364, Fat: 23.2, Fiber: 2.3g, Carbs: 5.1g, Protein: 35.4g

## Turkey With Lentils

Servings: 7    Cooking Time: 51 Minutes
**Ingredients:**
- 3 tablespoons olive oil, divided
- 1 onion, chopped
- 1 tablespoon fresh ginger, minced
- 4 garlic cloves, minced
- 3 plum tomatoes, chopped finely
- 2 cups dried red lentils, soaked for 30 minutes and drained
- 2 cups filtered water
- 2 teaspoons cumin seeds
- ½ teaspoon cayenne pepper
- 1 pound lean ground turkey
- 1 jalapeño pepper, seeded and chopped
- 2 scallions, chopped
- ¼ cup fresh cilantro, chopped

**Directions:**

In a Dutch oven, heat 1 tablespoon of oil over medium heat and sauté the onion, ginger and garlic for about 5 minutes. Stir in tomatoes, lentils and water and bring to a boil Now, reduce the heat to medium-low and simmer, covered for about 30 minutes. Meanwhile, in a skillet, heat remaining oil over medium heat and sauté the cumin seeds and cayenne pepper for about 1 minute. Transfer the mixture into a small bowl and set aside. In the same skillet, add turkey and cook for about 4-5 minutes. Add the jalapeño and scallion and cook for about 4-5 minutes. Add the spiced oil mixture and stir to combine well. Transfer the turkey mixture in simmering lentils and simmer for about 10-15 minutes or until desired doneness. Serve hot. Meal Prep Tip: Transfer the turkey mixture into a large bowl and set aside to cool. Divide the mixture into 4 containers evenly. Cover the containers and refrigerate for 1-2 days. Reheat in the microwave before serving.
**Nutrition Info:**Calories 361 Total Fat 11.5.4 g Saturated Fat 2.4 g Cholesterol 46 mg Total Carbs 37 g Sugar 3.4 g Fiber 18 g Sodium 937mg Potassium 331 mg Protein 27.9 g

## Chicken Cacciatore

Servings: 4      Cooking Time: 10 Minutes
**Ingredients:**
- 8 chicken drumsticks; bone-in
- 1/2 cup black olives; pitted and sliced
- 1 bay leaf
- 1 tsp. garlic powder
- 1 yellow onion; chopped
- 28 oz. canned tomatoes and juice; crushed
- 1 tsp. oregano; dried
- Salt and black pepper to the taste

**Directions:**
In a heat proof dish that fits your air fryer, mix chicken with salt, pepper, garlic powder, bay leaf, onion, tomatoes and juice, oregano and olives; toss, introduce in your preheated air fryer and cook at 365 °F, for 20 minutes. Divide among plates and serve.
**Nutrition Info:**Calories: 300; Fat: 12; Fiber: 8; Carbs: 20; Protein: 24

## Crock-pot Buffalo Chicken Dip

Servings: 10      Cooking Time: 3 Hours
**Ingredients:**
- 2 cups cooked chicken, chopped into small pieces
- 1 cup ranch dressing
- 16 oz cream cheese, cubed and softened
- 5 ounces' hot sauce

**Directions:**
add 5 oz hot sauce, 16 ounces cubed cream cheese, and 1 cup ranch dressing to a 3-quart Crock-Pot slow cooker. Cover it and cook for about 2 hours on Low, with occasional stirring. Once cheese is melted, add 2 cups of cooked chicken. Cover the Crock-Pot slow cooker again and cook again for 1 hour on Low. Serve buffalo chicken along with veggies or any of your favorite chips.
**Nutrition Info:**344 calories; 29 g fat; 5 g total carbs; 15 g protein

## Chicken & Tofu

Servings: 6      Cooking Time: 25 Minutes
**Ingredients:**
- 2 tablespoons olive oil, divided
- 2 tablespoons orange juice
- 1 tablespoon Worcestershire sauce
- 1 tablespoon low-sodium soy sauce
- 1 teaspoon ground turmeric
- 1 teaspoon dry mustard
- 8 oz. chicken breast, cooked and sliced into cubes
- 8 oz. extra-firm tofu, drained and sliced into cubed
- 2 carrots, sliced into thin strips
- 1 cup mushroom, sliced
- 2 cups fresh bean sprouts
- 3 green onions, sliced
- 1 red sweet pepper, sliced into strips

**Directions:**
In a bowl, mix half of the oil with the orange juice, Worcestershire sauce, soy sauce, turmeric and mustard. Coat all sides of chicken and tofu with the sauce. Marinate for 1 hour. In a pan over medium heat, add 1 tablespoon oil. Add carrot and cook for 2 minutes. Add mushroom and cook for another 2 minutes. Add bean sprouts, green onion and sweet pepper. Cook for two to three minutes. Stir in the chicken and heat through.
**Nutrition Info:**Calories 285 Total Fat 9 g Saturated Fat 1 g Cholesterol 32 mg Sodium 331 mg Total Carbohydrate 30 g Dietary Fiber 4 g Total Sugars 4 g Protein 20 g Potassium 559 mg

## Peppered Broccoli Chicken

Servings: 4      Cooking Time: 30 Minutes
**Ingredients:**
- 1 tbsp Sage (sliced)
- 1 cup Broccoli florets
- 1 lb. (no bones and skin) Chicken breast
- 3 pieces Garlic cloves
- 1 cup Tomato passata
- What you'll need from the store cupboard:
- Salt and Black pepper to taste
- 2 tbsp. Olive oil

**Directions:**
Put the instant pot on Sauté option, then put the oil and cook it. After that, put the chicken and garlic then heats it for 5 minutes. Put the other ingredients, then cover it and heat it for 25 minutes on high temperature. Release the pressure gradually for 10 minutes then split them among your plates before eating.
**Nutrition Info:**Calories: 217, Fat: 10.1g, Fiber: 1.8g, Carbs: 5.9g, Protein: 25.4g

## Peppered Chicken Breast With Basil

Servings: 4      Cooking Time: 20 Minutes
**Ingredients:**
- ¼ cup Red bell peppers
- 1 cup Chicken stock
- 2 pieces (no skin and bones) Chicken breasts
- 4 pieces Garlic cloves (crushed)

- 1 and a half tbsp Basil (crushed)
- What you'll need from the store cupboard:
- 1 tbsp Chili powder

**Directions:**
In the instant pot, combine the ingredients then cover them and cook for 25 minutes on high temperature. Release the pressure quickly for 5 minutes then split them among your plates before eating.
**Nutrition Info:** Calories: 230, Fat: 12.4g, Fiber: 0.8g, Carbs: 2.7g, Protein: 33.2g

## Spicy Chicken Drumsticks

Servings: 6     Cooking Time: 10 Minutes
**Ingredients:**
- 1/2 cup ketchup
- 1/4 cup dark brown sugar
- 1/4 cup red wine vinegar
- 3 tablespoon soy sauce
- 1 tablespoon chicken seasoning
- Salt to taste
- 6 chicken drumsticks

**Directions:**
Combine ketchup, brown sugar, red wine vinegar, soy sauce, seasoning, and salt in the Instant Pot. Add chicken pieces and stir to coat.     Close Instant Pot Lid, and make sure steam release handle is in the 'Sealing' position.     Cook on 'Manual' (or 'Pressure Cook') for 12 minutes.     Do a quick release of pressure and carefully open the Instant Pot.     Remove chicken pieces and set aside.     Press 'Saute' and cook the sauce thickened, about 5 to 7 minutes.
**Nutrition Info:** Calories 145 Fat 28 g Carbohydrates 13.6 g Sugar 2 g Protein 4.9 g Cholesterol 45 mg

## Crock Pot Chicken Cacciatore

Servings: 6     Cooking Time: 4 Hours
**Ingredients:**
- 1 can (14.5 oz) tomatoes, diced
- 6 medium chicken thighs, skins removed
- 1 onion, sliced
- 1 tablespoon Italian seasoning
- 1 green bell pepper, seeded and sliced
- 3 clove garlic, minced
- 2 can (6-oz, no salt added) tomato paste

**Directions:**
To a Crock-Pot slow cooker, add all ingredients and cook for 4 hours on High.     Once done, serve chicken cacciatore with whole wheat rotini pasta, if desired.
**Nutrition Info:** 170 calories; 5 g fat; 18 g total carbs; 16 g protein

## Chicken Cabbage Curry

Servings: 4     Cooking Time: 30 Minutes
**Ingredients:**
- 1 kg of boneless chicken, cut into small pieces
- 2 cans of coconut milk
- 3 tablespoons of curry paste
- 1 small onion, diced
- 1 medium red bell pepper
- 1 medium green bell pepper

- 1/2 head of a big cabbage

**Directions:**
Dissolve the curry paste into the coconut milk and stir well. Pour into the Instant Pot.     Add the chicken to the coconut curry mixture.     Chop both peppers into cubes and add to the pot.     Add the onion.     Cut the cabbage into slices and add to the pot. Make sure all the ingredients are coated with coconut milk.     Put the lid on, seal and cook on Low for 30 minutes.     When it's cooked, open carefully and serve immediately.
**Nutrition Info:** Calories 301 Fat 27.2 g Carbohydrates 13.6 g Sugar 6 g Protein 4.9 g Cholesterol 33 mg

## Crock-pot Slow Cooker Chicken & Sweet Potatoes

Servings: 4     Cooking Time: 5-7 Hours
**Ingredients:**
- 1 1/2 cup low-sodium and low-fat chicken broth
- 1 bay leave
- 4 (4 oz) chicken thighs, skinless and boneless
- 2 tablespoons Dijon mustard
- 1 onion, chopped
- 1/4 teaspoon dried thyme
- 2 large sweet potatoes, peeled and sliced into large rounds
- 3 tablespoons Splenda Brown Sugar blend

**Directions:**
Place 4 (4 oz) chicken thighs into the Crock-Pot slow cooker.     Top chicken thighs with sliced potatoes and chopped onions.     Now add all leftover ingredients to the Crock-Pot slow cooker. Cook for about 5-7 hours on low until chicken is completely cooked through.     Once done, remove bay leaf from the Crock-Pot slow cooker. Serve right away.
**Nutrition Info:** 75 calories; 7 g fat; 32 g total carbs; 21 g protein

## Chicken And Asparagus

Servings: 4     Cooking Time: 10 Minutes
**Ingredients:**
- 8 chicken wings; halved
- 8 asparagus spears
- 1 tbsp. rosemary; chopped
- 1 tsp. cumin; ground
- Salt and black pepper to the taste

**Directions:**
Pat dry chicken wings, season with salt, pepper, cumin and rosemary, put them in your air fryer's basket and cook at 360 °F, for 20 minutes.     Meanwhile; heat up a pan over medium heat, add asparagus, add water to cover, steam for a few minutes; transfer to a bowl filled with ice water, drain and arrange on plates. Add chicken wings on the side and serve.
**Nutrition Info:** Calories: 270; Fat: 8; Fiber: 12; Carbs: 24; Protein: 22

## Fried Lemon Chicken

Servings: 6     Cooking Time: 20 Minutes.
**Ingredients:**
- 6 chicken thighs

- 2 tbsp. olive oil
- 2 tbsp. lemon juice
- 1 tbsp. Italian herbal seasoning mix
- 1 tsp. Celtic sea salt
- 1 tsp. ground fresh pepper
- 1 lemon, thinly slice

**Directions:**
Add all ingredients, except sliced lemon, to bowl or bag, stir to cover chicken.    Let marinate for 30 minutes overnight.    Remove the chicken and let the excess oil drip (it does not need to dry out, just do not drip with tons of excess oil).    Arrange the chicken thighs and the lemon slices in the fryer basket, being careful not to push the chicken thighs too close to each other.    Set the fryer to 200 degrees and cook for 10 minutes.    Remove the basket from the fryer and turn the chicken thighs to the other side.    Cook again at 200 for another 10 minutes.
**Nutrition Info:**Calories: 215 Fat: 13g Carbohydrates: 1g Protein: 2 Sugar: 1g Cholesterol: 130mg

## Mustard And Maple Turkey Breast

Servings: 6      Cooking Time: 1 Hr
**Ingredients:**
- 5 lb of whole turkey breast
- ¼ cup maple syrup
- 2 tbsp dijon mustard
- ½ tbsp smoked paprika
- 1 tbsp thyme
- 2 tbsp olive oil
- ½ tbsp sage
- ½ tbsp salt and black pepper
- 1 tbsp butter, melted

**Directions:**
Preheat the Air fryer to 350 F and brush the turkey with the olive oil. Combine all herbs and seasoning, in a small bowl, and rub the turkey with the mixture. Air fry the turkey for 25 minutes. Flip the turkey on its side and continue to cook for 12 more minutes.    Now, turn on the opposite side, and again, cook for an additional 12 minutes. Whisk the butter, maple and mustard together in a small bowl. When done, brush the glaze all over the turkey. Return to the air fryer and cook for 5 more minutes, until nice and crispy.
**Nutrition Info:**Calories: 529; Carbs: 77g; Fat: 20g; Protein: 13g

## Dry Rub Chicken Wings

Servings: 4      Cooking Time: 30 Minutes
**Ingredients:**
- 9g garlic powder
- 1 cube of chicken broth, reduced sodium
- 5g of salt
- 3g black pepper
- 1g smoked paprika
- 1g cayenne pepper
- 3g Old Bay seasoning, sodium free
- 3g onion powder
- 1g dried oregano
- 453g chicken wings
- Nonstick Spray Oil
- Ranch sauce, to serve

**Directions:**
Preheat the air fryer. Set the temperature to 180 °C. Put ingredients in a bowl and mix well.    Season the chicken wings with half the seasoning mixture and sprinkle abundantly with oil spray.    Place the chicken wings in the preheated air fryer.    Select Chicken, set the timer to 30 minutes.    Shake the baskets halfway through cooking.
**Nutrition Info:**Calories: 120 Fat: 6g Carbohydrates 0g Protein: 18g Sugar: 0g

# Fish And Seafood Recipes

## Grilled Tuna Steaks

Servings: 6     Cooking Time: 10 Minutes,
**Ingredients:**
- 6 6 oz. tuna steaks
- 3 tbsp. fresh basil, diced
- What you'll need from store cupboard:
- 4 ½ tsp olive oil
- ¾ tsp salt
- ¼ tsp pepper
- Nonstick cooking spray

**Directions:**
Heat grill to medium heat. Spray rack with cooking spray. Drizzle both sides of the tuna with oil. Sprinkle with basil, salt and pepper.     Place on grill and cook 5 minutes per side, tuna should be slightly pink in the center. Serve.
**Nutrition Info:**Calories 343 Total Carbs 0g Protein 51g Fat 14g Sugar 0g Fiber 0g

## Delicious Fish Tacos

Servings: 8     Cooking Time: 8 Minutes
**Ingredients:**
- 4 tilapia fillets
- 1/4 cup fresh cilantro, chopped
- 1/4 cup fresh lime juice
- 2 tbsp paprika
- 1 tbsp olive oil
- Pepper
- Salt

**Directions:**
Pour 2 cups of water into the instant pot then place steamer rack in the pot.     Place fish fillets on parchment paper.     Season fish fillets with paprika, pepper, and salt and drizzle with oil and lime juice.     Fold parchment paper around the fish fillets and place them on a steamer rack in the pot.     Seal pot with lid and cook on high for 8 minutes.     Once done, release pressure using quick release. Remove lid.     Remove fish packet from pot and open it.     Shred the fish with a fork and serve.
**Nutrition Info:**Calories 67 Fat 2.5 g Carbohydrates 1.1 g Sugar 0.2 g Protein 10.8 g Cholesterol 28 mg

## Shrimp Coconut Curry

Servings: 2     Cooking Time: 20 Minutes
**Ingredients:**
- 0.5lb cooked shrimp
- 1 thinly sliced onion
- 1 cup coconut yogurt
- 3tbsp curry paste
- 1tbsp oil or ghee

**Directions:**
Set the Instant Pot to sauté and add the onion, oil, and curry paste.     When the onion is soft, add the remaining ingredients and seal.     Cook on Stew for 20 minutes.     Release the pressure naturally.

**Nutrition Info:**Calories: 380 Carbs 13; Sugar 4; Fat 22; Protein 40; GL 14

## Salmon & Shrimp Stew

Servings: 6     Cooking Time: 21 Minutes
**Ingredients:**
- 2 tablespoons olive oil
- ½ cup onion, chopped finely
- 2 garlic cloves, minced
- 1 Serrano pepper, chopped
- 1 teaspoon smoked paprika
- 4 cups fresh tomatoes, chopped
- 4 cups low-sodium chicken broth
- 1 pound salmon fillets, cubed
- 1 pound shrimp, peeled and deveined
- 2 tablespoons fresh lime juice
- ¼ cup fresh basil, chopped
- ¼ cup fresh parsley, chopped
- Ground black pepper, as required
- 2 scallions, chopped

**Directions:**
In a large soup pan, melt coconut oil over medium-high heat and sauté the onion for about 5-6 minutes.     Add the garlic, Serrano pepper and smoked paprika and sauté for about 1 minute.     Add the tomatoes and broth and bring to a gentle simmer over medium heat.     Simmer for about 5 minutes.     Add the salmon and simmer for about 3-4 minutes.     Stir in the remaining seafood and cook for about 4-5 minutes.     Stir in the lemon juice, basil, parsley, sea salt and black pepper and remove from heat.     Serve hot with the garnishing of scallion. Meal Prep Tip: Transfer the stew into a large bowl and set aside to cool. Divide the stew into 4 containers evenly. Cover the containers and refrigerate for 1-2 days. Reheat in the microwave before serving.
**Nutrition Info:**Calories 271 Total Fat 11 g Saturated Fat 1.8 g Cholesterol 193 mg Total Carbs 8.6 g Sugar 3.8 g Fiber 2.1 g Sodium 273 mg Potassium 763 mg Protein 34.7 g

## Swordfish With Tomato Salsa

Servings: 4     Cooking Time: 12 Minutes
**Ingredients:**
- 1 cup tomato, chopped
- ¼ cup tomatillo, chopped
- 2 tablespoons fresh cilantro, chopped
- ¼ cup avocado, chopped
- 1 clove garlic, minced
- 1 jalapeño pepper, chopped
- 1 tablespoon lime juice
- Salt and pepper to taste
- 4 swordfish steaks
- 1 clove garlic, sliced in half
- 2 tablespoons lemon juice
- ½ teaspoon ground cumin

**Directions:**
Preheat your grill.     In a bowl, mix the tomato, tomatillo, cilantro, avocado, garlic, jalapeño, lime juice,

salt and pepper. Cover the bowl with foil and put in the refrigerator. Rub each swordfish steak with sliced garlic. Drizzle lemon juice on both sides. Season with salt, pepper and cumin. Grill for 12 minutes or until the fish is fully cooked. Serve with salsa.

**Nutrition Info:** Calories 125 g Fat 27.2 g Carbohydrates 13.6 g Protein 7 g Cholesterol 31 mg

## Shrimp Boil

Servings: 4    Cooking Time: 15 Minutes

**Ingredients:**
- 8 oz. raw shrimp, unpeeled
- 8 ooz. chicken sausage, small 1 inch pieces
- 8 oz. baby potatoes
- 1 sliced leek
- 2 corns, cut into half
- What you will need from the store cupboard:
- 3 tablespoons lemon juice
- 10 cups of water
- ¼ cup Old Bay seasoning
- Melted butter
- Lemon wedges

**Directions:**
Bring together the lemon juice, Old Bay, and water in your pot. Boil. Include potatoes and cook for 5-7 minutes. Add the sausage, shrimp, leek, and corn. Cook while stirring for another 5 minutes. The vegetables should be tender and the shrimp must be pink. Now divide the vegetables, sausage, and shrimp with spoon and tongs among the serving bowls. Drizzle the cooking liquid equally. Serve with butter (optional).

**Nutrition Info:** Calories 202, Carbohydrates 22g, Fiber 2g, Sugar 0g, Cholesterol 109mg, Total Fat 5g, Protein 19g

## Shrimp & Artichoke Skillet

Servings: 4    Cooking Time: 10 Minutes

**Ingredients:**
- 1 ½ cups shrimp, peel & devein
- 2 shallots, diced
- 1 tbsp. margarine
- What you'll need from store cupboard
- 2 12 oz. jars artichoke hearts, drain & rinse
- 2 cups white wine
- 2 cloves garlic, diced fine

**Directions:**
Melt margarine in a large skillet over med-high heat. Add shallot and garlic and cook until they start to brown, stirring frequently. Add artichokes and cook 5 minutes. Reduce heat and add wine. Cook 3 minutes, stirring occasionally. Add the shrimp and cook just until they turn pink. Serve.

**Nutrition Info:** Calories 487 Total Carbs 26g Net Carbs 17g Protein 64g Fat 5g Sugar 3g Fiber 9g

## Red Clam Sauce & Pasta

Servings: 4    Cooking Time: 3 Hours,

**Ingredients:**
- 1 onion, diced
- ¼ cup fresh parsley, diced

- What you'll need from store cupboard:
- 2 6 ½ oz. cans clams, chopped, undrained
- 14 ½ oz. tomatoes, diced, undrained
- 6 oz. tomato paste
- 2 cloves garlic, diced
- 1 bay leaf
- 1 tbsp. sunflower oil
- 1 tsp Splenda
- 1 tsp basil
- ½ tsp thyme
- ½ Homemade Pasta, cook & drain (chapter 15)

**Directions:**
Heat oil in a small skillet over med-high heat. Add onion and cook until tender, Add garlic and cook 1 minute more. Transfer to crock pot. Add remaining Ingredients, except pasta, cover and cook on low 3-4 hours. Discard bay leaf and serve over cooked pasta.

**Nutrition Info:** Calories 223 Total Carbs 32g Net Carbs 27g Protein 12g Fat 6g Sugar 15g Fiber 5g

## Grilled Herbed Salmon With Raspberry Sauce & Cucumber Dill Dip

Servings: 4    Cooking Time: 30 Minutes

**Ingredients:**
- 3 salmon fillets
- 1 tablespoon olive oil
- Salt and pepper to taste
- 1 teaspoon fresh sage, chopped
- 1 tablespoon fresh parsley, chopped
- 2 tablespoons apple juice
- 1 cup raspberries
- 1 teaspoon Worcestershire sauce
- 1 cup cucumber, chopped
- 2 tablespoons light mayonnaise
- ½ teaspoon dried dill

**Directions:**
Coat the salmon fillets with oil. Season with salt, pepper, sage and parsley. Cover the salmon with foil. Grill for 20 minutes or until fish is flaky. While waiting, mix the apple juice, raspberries and Worcestershire sauce. Pour the mixture into a saucepan over medium heat. Bring to a boil and then simmer for 8 minutes. In another bowl, mix the rest of the ingredients. Serve salmon with raspberry sauce and cucumber dip.

**Nutrition Info:** Calories 256 Total Fat 15 g Saturated Fat 3 g Cholesterol 68 mg Sodium 176 mg Total Carbohydrate 6 g Dietary Fiber 1 g Total Sugars 5 g Protein 23 g Potassium 359 mg

## Shrimp With Green Beans

Servings: 4    Cooking Time: 2 Minutes

**Ingredients:**
- ¾ pound fresh green beans, trimmed
- 1 pound medium frozen shrimp, peeled and deveined
- 2 tablespoons fresh lemon juice
- 2 tablespoons olive oil
- Salt and ground black pepper, as required

**Directions:**

Arrange a steamer trivet in the Instant Pot and pour cup of water.    Arrange the green beans on top of trivet in a single layer and top with shrimp.    Drizzle with oil and lemon juice.    Sprinkle with salt and black pepper. Close the lid and place the pressure valve to "Seal" position.    Press "Steam" and just use the default time of 2 minutes.    Press "Cancel" and allow a "Natural" release.    Open the lid and serve.
**Nutrition Info:**Calories: 223, Fats: 1g, Carbs: 7.9g, Sugar: 1.4g, Proteins: 27.4g, Sodium: 322mg

## Crab Curry

Servings: 2    Cooking Time: 20 Minutes
**Ingredients:**
- 0.5lb chopped crab
- 1 thinly sliced red onion
- 0.5 cup chopped tomato
- 3tbsp curry paste
- 1tbsp oil or ghee

**Directions:**
Set the Instant Pot to sauté and add the onion, oil, and curry paste.    When the onion is soft, add the remaining ingredients and seal.    Cook on Stew for 20 minutes.    Release the pressure naturally.
**Nutrition Info:**Calories 2; Carbs 11; Sugar 4; Fat 10; Protein 24; GL 9

## Mussels In Tomato Sauce

Servings: 4    Cooking Time: 3 Minutes
**Ingredients:**
- 2 tomatoes, seeded and chopped finely
- 2 pounds mussels, scrubbed and de-bearded
- 1 cup low-sodium chicken broth
- 1 tablespoon fresh lemon juice
- 2 garlic cloves, minced

**Directions:**
In the pot of Instant Pot, place tomatoes, garlic, wine and bay leaf and stir to combine.    Arrange the mussels on top.    Close the lid and place the pressure valve to "Seal" position.    Press "Manual" and cook under "High Pressure" for about 3 minutes.    Press "Cancel" and carefully allow a "Quick" release.    Open the lid and serve hot.
**Nutrition Info:**Calories 213, Fats 25.2g, Carbs 11g, Sugar 1. Proteins 28.2g, Sodium 670mg

## Shrimp Salad

Servings: 6    Cooking Time: 4 Minutes
**Ingredients:**
- For Salad:
- 1 pound shrimp, peeled and deveined
- Salt and ground black pepper, as required
- 1 teaspoon olive oil
- 1½ cups carrots, peeled and julienned
- 1½ cups red cabbage, shredded
- 1½ cup cucumber, julienned
- 5 cups fresh baby arugula
- ¼ cup fresh basil, chopped
- ¼ cup fresh cilantro, chopped
- 4 cups lettuce, torn

- ¼ cup almonds, chopped
- For Dressing:
- 2 tablespoons natural almond butter
- 1 garlic clove, crushed
- 1 tablespoon fresh cilantro, chopped
- 1 tablespoon fresh lime juice
- 1 tablespoon unsweetened applesauce
- 2 teaspoons balsamic vinegar
- ½ teaspoon cayenne pepper
- Salt, as required
- 1 tablespoon water
- 1/3 cup olive oil

**Directions:**
Slowly, add the oil, beating continuously until smooth. For salad: in a bowl, add shrimp, salt, black pepper and oil and toss to coat well.    Heat a skillet over medium-high heat and cook the shrimp for about 2 minutes per side.    Remove from the heat and set aside to cool.    In a large bowl, add the shrimp, vegetables and mix well. For dressing: in a bowl, add all ingredients except oil and beat until well combined.    Place the dressing over shrimp mixture and gently, toss to coat well.    Serve immediately.    Meal Prep Tip: Divide dressing in 6 large mason jars evenly. Place the remaining ingredients in the layers of carrots, followed by cabbage, cucumber, arugula, basil, cilantro, shrimp, lettuce and almonds. Cover each jar with the lid tightly and refrigerate for about 1 day. Shake the jars well just before serving.
**Nutrition Info:**Calories 274 Total Fat 17.7 g Saturated Fat 2.4 g Cholesterol 159 mg Total Carbs 10 g Sugar 3.8 g Fiber 2.9 g Sodium 242 mg Potassium 481 mg Protein 20.5 g

## Grilled Herbed Salmon With Raspberry Sauce & Cucumber Dill Dip

Servings: 4    Cooking Time: 30 Minutes
**Ingredients:**
- 3 salmon fillets
- 1 tablespoon olive oil
- Salt and pepper to taste
- 1 teaspoon fresh sage, chopped
- 1 tablespoon fresh parsley, chopped
- 2 tablespoons apple juice
- 1 cup raspberries
- 1 teaspoon Worcestershire sauce
- 1 cup cucumber, chopped
- 2 tablespoons light mayonnaise
- ½ teaspoon dried dill

**Directions:**
Coat the salmon fillets with oil.    Season with salt, pepper, sage and parsley.    Cover the salmon with foil. Grill for 20 minutes or until fish is flaky.    While waiting, mix the apple juice, raspberries and Worcestershire sauce.    Pour the mixture into a saucepan over medium heat.    Bring to a boil and then simmer for 8 minutes.    In another bowl, mix the rest of the ingredients.    Serve salmon with raspberry sauce and cucumber dip.
**Nutrition Info:**Calories 301 Fat 27.2 g Carbohydrates 13.6 g Protein 4.9 g Cholesterol 33 mg

## Cajun Shrimp & Roasted Vegetables

Servings: 4    Cooking Time: 15 Minutes
**Ingredients:**
- 1 lb. large shrimp, peeled and deveined
- 2 zucchinis, sliced
- 2 yellow squash, sliced
- ½ bunch asparagus, cut into thirds
- 2 red bell pepper, cut into chunks
- What you'll need from store cupboard:
- 2 tbsp. olive oil
- 2 tbsp. Cajun Seasoning
- Salt & pepper, to taste

**Directions:**
Heat oven to 400 degrees.    Combine shrimp and vegetables in a large bowl. Add oil and seasoning and toss to coat.    Spread evenly in a large baking sheet and bake 15-20 minutes, or until vegetables are tender. Serve.
**Nutrition Info:**Calories 251 Total Carbs 13g Net Carbs 9g Protein 30g Fat 9g Sugar 6g Fiber 4g

## Parmesan Herb Fish

Servings: 4    Cooking Time: 15 Minutes
**Ingredients:**
- 16 oz. tilapia fillets
- 1/3 cup almonds, sliced and chopped
- ½ teaspoon parsley, chopped
- ¼ cup dry bread crumbs
- What you will need from the store cupboard:
- ½ teaspoon garlic powder
- ¼ teaspoon black pepper, ground
- ½ teaspoon paprika
- 3 tablespoons Parmesan cheese, grated
- Olive oil

**Directions:**
Preheat your oven to 350 °F.    Mix the bread crumbs, almonds, seasonings and Parmesan cheese in a dish. Brush oil lightly on the fish.    Coat the almond mix evenly.    Now keep the fish on a greased foil-lined baking pan.    Bake for 10-12 minutes. The fish should flake easily with your fork.
**Nutrition Info:**Calories 225, Carbohydrates 7g, Fiber 1g, Cholesterol 57mg, Total Fat 9g, Protein 29g, Sodium 202mg

## Lemony Salmon

Servings: 3    Cooking Time: 3 Minutes
**Ingredients:**
- 1 pound salmon fillet, cut into 3 pieces
- 3 teaspoons fresh dill, chopped
- 5 tablespoons fresh lemon juice, divided
- Salt and ground black pepper, as required

**Directions:**
Arrange a steamer trivet in Instant Pot and pour ¼ cup of lemon juice.    Season the salmon with salt and black pepper evenly.    Place the salmon pieces on top of trivet, skin side down and drizzle with remaining lemon juice. Now, sprinkle the salmon pieces with dill evenly. Close the lid and place the pressure valve to "Seal" position.    Press "Steam" and use the default time of 3

minutes.    Press "Cancel" and allow a "Natural" release. Open the lid and serve hot.
**Nutrition Info:**Calories: 20 Fats: 9.6g, Carbs: 1.1g, Sugar: 0.5g, Proteins: 29.7g, Sodium: 74mg

## Herring & Veggies Soup

Servings: 5    Cooking Time: 25 Minutes
**Ingredients:**
- 2 tablespoons olive oil
- 1 shallot, chopped
- 2 small garlic cloves, minced
- 1 jalapeño pepper, chopped
- 1 head cabbage, chopped
- 1 small red bell pepper, seeded and chopped finely
- 1 small yellow bell pepper, seeded and chopped finely
- 5 cups low-sodium chicken broth
- 2 (4-ounce) boneless herring fillets, cubed
- ¼ cup fresh cilantro, minced
- 2 tablespoons fresh lemon juice
- Ground black pepper, as required
- 2 scallions, chopped

**Directions:**
In a large soup pan, heat the oil over medium heat and sauté shallot and garlic for 2-3 minutes.    Add the cabbage and bell peppers and sauté for about 3-4 minutes.    Add the broth and bring to a boil over high heat.    Now, reduce the heat to medium-low and simmer for about 10 minutes.    Add the herring cubes and cook for about 5-6 minutes.    Stir in the cilantro, lemon juice, salt and black pepper and cook for about 1-2 minutes.    Serve hot with the topping of scallion. Meal Prep Tip: Transfer the soup into a large bowl and set aside to cool. Divide the soup into 5 containers evenly. Cover the containers and refrigerate for 1-2 days. Reheat in the microwave before serving.
**Nutrition Info:**Calories 215 Total Fat 11.2g Saturated Fat 2.1 g Cholesterol 35 mg Total Carbs 14.7 g Sugar 7 g Fiber 4.5 g Sodium 152 mg Potassium 574 mg Protein 15.1 g

## Garlicky Clams

Servings: 4    Cooking Time: 5 Minutes
**Ingredients:**
- 3 lbs clams, clean
- 4 garlic cloves
- 1/4 cup olive oil
- 1/2 cup fresh lemon juice
- 1 cup white wine
- Pepper
- Salt

**Directions:**
Add oil into the inner pot of instant pot and set the pot on sauté mode.    Add garlic and sauté for 1 minute. Add wine and cook for 2 minutes.    Add remaining ingredients and stir well.    Seal pot with lid and cook on high for 2 minutes.    Once done, allow to release pressure naturally. Remove lid.    Serve and enjoy.
**Nutrition Info:**Calories 332 Fat 13.5 g Carbohydrates 40.5 g Sugar 12.4 g Protein 2.5 g Cholesterol 0 mg

## Tuna Salad

Servings: 2

**Ingredients:**
- 2 (5-ounce) cans water packed tuna, drained
- 2 tablespoons fat-free plain Greek yogurt
- Salt and ground black pepper, as required
- 2 medium carrots, peeled and shredded
- 2 apples, cored and chopped
- 2 cups fresh spinach, torn

**Directions:**
In a large bowl, add the tuna, yogurt, salt and black pepper and gently, stir to combine.      Add the carrots and apples and stir to combine.      Serve immediately. Meal Prep Tip: Divide tuna mixture in 2 mason jars evenly. Place the remaining ingredients in the layers of, carrots, apples and spinach. Cover each jar with the lid tightly and refrigerate for about 1 day. Shake the jars well just before serving.

**Nutrition Info:**Calories 306 Total Fat 1.8g Saturated Fat 0 g Cholesterol 63 mg Total Carbs 38 g Sugar 26 g Fiber 7.6 g Sodium 324 mg Potassium 602 mg Protein 35.8 g

## Grilled Tuna Salad

Servings: 4      Cooking Time: 15 Minutes

**Ingredients:**
- 4 oz. tuna fish, 4 steaks
- ¾ lb. red potatoes, diced
- ½ lb. green beans, trimmed
- 16 kalamata olives, chopped
- 4 cups of baby spinach leaves
- What you will need from the store cupboard:
- 2 tablespoons canola oil
- 2 tablespoons red wine vinegar
- 1/8 teaspoon salt
- 1 tablespoon water
- 1/8 teaspoon red pepper flakes

**Directions:**
Steam the green beans and potatoes to make them tender.      Drain, rinse to shake off the excess water. Bring together the vinaigrette ingredients in your jar while the vegetables are cooking. Close the lid and shake well. Everything should blend well.      Brush the vinaigrette over your fish.      Coat canola oil on your pan. Heat over medium temperature.      Grill each side of the tuna for 3 minutes.      Now divide the greens on your serving plates.      Arrange the green beans, olives, and potatoes over the greens.      Drizzle the vinaigrette on the salad. Top with tuna.

**Nutrition Info:**Calories 345, Carbohydrates 26g, Fiber 5g, Cholesterol 40mg, Total Fat 14g, Protein 29g, Sodium 280mg

## Mediterranean Fish Fillets

Servings: 4      Cooking Time: 3 Minutes

**Ingredients:**
- 4 cod fillets
- 1 lb grape tomatoes, halved
- 1 cup olives, pitted and sliced
- 2 tbsp capers
- 1 tsp dried thyme
- 2 tbsp olive oil
- 1 tsp garlic, minced
- Pepper
- Salt

**Directions:**
Pour 1 cup water into the instant pot then place steamer rack in the pot.      Spray heat-safe baking dish with cooking spray.      Add half grape tomatoes into the dish and season with pepper and salt.      Arrange fish fillets on top of cherry tomatoes. Drizzle with oil and season with garlic, thyme, capers, pepper, and salt.      Spread olives and remaining grape tomatoes on top of fish fillets. Place dish on top of steamer rack in the pot.      Seal pot with a lid and select manual and cook on high for 3 minutes.      Once done, release pressure using quick release. Remove lid.      Serve and enjoy.

**Nutrition Info:**Calories 212 Fat 11.9 g Carbohydrates 7.1 g Sugar 3 g Protein 21.4 g Cholesterol 55 mg

## Herbed Salmon

Servings: 4      Cooking Time: 3 Minutes

**Ingredients:**
- 4 (4-ounce) salmon fillets
- ¼ cup olive oil
- 2 tablespoons fresh lemon juice
- 1 garlic clove, minced
- ¼ teaspoon dried oregano
- Salt and ground black pepper, as required
- 4 fresh rosemary sprigs
- 4 lemon slices

**Directions:**
For dressing: in a large bowl, add oil, lemon juice, garlic, oregano, salt and black pepper and beat until well co combined.      Arrange a steamer trivet in the Instant Pot and pour 11/2 cups of water in Instant Pot.      Place the salmon fillets on top of trivet in a single layer and top with dressing.      Arrange 1 rosemary sprig and 1 lemon slice over each fillet.      Close the lid and place the pressure valve to "Seal" position.      Press "Steam" and just use the default time of 3 minutes.      Press "Cancel" and carefully allow a "Quick" release.      Open the lid and serve hot.

**Nutrition Info:**Calories 262, Fats 17g, Carbs 0.7g, Sugar 0.2g, Proteins 22.1g, Sodium 91mg

## Tarragon Scallops

Servings: 4      Cooking Time: 15 Minutes

**Ingredients:**
- 1 cup water
- 1 lb. asparagus spears, trimmed
- 2 lemons
- 1 ¼ lb. scallops
- Salt and pepper to taste
- 1 tablespoon olive oil
- 1 tablespoon fresh tarragon, chopped

**Directions:**
Pour water into a pot.      Bring to a boil.      Add asparagus spears.      Cover and cook for 5 minutes. Drain and transfer to a plate.      Slice one lemon into

wedges. Squeeze juice and shred zest from the remaining lemon. Season the scallops with salt and pepper. Put a pan over medium heat. Add oil to the pan. Cook the scallops until golden brown. Transfer to the same plate, putting scallops beside the asparagus. Add lemon zest, juice and tarragon to the pan. Cook for 1 minute. Drizzle tarragon sauce over the scallops and asparagus.

**Nutrition Info:**Calories 250 g Fat 10 g Carbohydrates 30 g Protein 15 g Cholesterol 24 mg

## Sardine Curry

Servings: 2     Cooking Time: 35 Minutes
**Ingredients:**
- 5 tins of sardines in tomato
- 1lb chopped vegetables
- 1 cup low sodium fish broth
- 3tbsp curry paste

**Directions:**
Mix all the ingredients in your Instant Pot. Cook on Stew for 35 minutes. Release the pressure naturally.

**Nutrition Info:**Calories 320; Carbs 8; Sugar 2; Fat 16; Protein GL 3

## Grilled Salmon With Ginger Sauce

Servings: 4     Cooking Time: 8 Minutes
**Ingredients:**
- 1 tablespoon toasted sesame oil
- 1 tablespoon fresh cilantro, chopped
- 1 tablespoon lime juice
- 1 teaspoon fish sauce
- 1 clove garlic, mashed
- 1 teaspoon fresh ginger, grated
- 1 teaspoon jalapeño pepper, minced
- 4 salmon fillets
- 1 tablespoon olive oil
- Salt and pepper to taste

**Directions:**
In a bowl, mix the sesame oil, cilantro, lime juice, fish sauce, garlic, ginger and jalapeño pepper. Preheat your grill. Brush oil on salmon. Season both sides with salt and pepper. Grill salmon for 6 to 8 minutes, turning once or twice. Take 1 tablespoon from the oil mixture. Brush this on the salmon while grilling. Serve grilled salmon with the remaining sauce.

**Nutrition Info:**Calories 204 Total Fat 11 g Saturated Fat 2 g Cholesterol 53 mg Sodium 320 mg Total Carbohydrate 2 g Dietary Fiber 0 g Total Sugars 2 g Protein 23 g Potassium 437 mg

## Shrimp With Broccoli

Servings: 6     Cooking Time: 12 Minutes
**Ingredients:**
- 2 tablespoons olive oil, divided
- 4 cups broccoli, chopped
- 2-3 tablespoons filtered water
- 1½ pounds large shrimp, peeled and deveined
- 2 garlic cloves, minced
- 1 (1-inch) piece fresh ginger, minced
- Salt and ground black pepper, as required

**Directions:**
In a large skillet, heat 1 tablespoon of oil over medium-high heat and cook the broccoli for about 1-2 minutes stirring continuously. Stir in the water and cook, covered for about 3-4 minutes, stirring occasionally. With a spoon, push the broccoli to side of the pan. Add the remaining oil and let it heat. Add the shrimp and cook for about 1-2 minutes, tossing occasionally. Add the remaining ingredients and sauté for about 2-3 minutes. Serve hot. Meal Prep Tip: Transfer the shrimp mixture into a large bowl and set aside to cool. Divide the shrimp mixture into 6 containers evenly. Cover the containers and refrigerate for 1 day. Reheat in the microwave before serving.

**Nutrition Info:**Calories 197 Total Fat 6.8 g Saturated Fat 1.3 g Cholesterol 239 mg Total Carbs 6.1 g Sugar 1.1 g Fiber 1.6 g Sodium 324 mg Potassium 389 mg Protein 27.6 g

## Citrus Salmon

Servings: 4     Cooking Time: 7 Minutes
**Ingredients:**
- 4 (4-ounce) salmon fillets
- 1 cup low-sodium chicken broth
- 1 teaspoon fresh ginger, minced
- 2 teaspoons fresh orange zest, grated finely
- 3 tablespoons fresh orange juice
- 1 tablespoon olive oil
- Ground black pepper, as required

**Directions:**
In Instant Pot, add all ingredients and mix. Close the lid and place the pressure valve to "Seal" position. Press "Manual" and cook under "High Pressure" for about 7 minutes. Press "Cancel" and allow a "Natural" release. Open the lid and serve the salmon fillets with the topping of cooking sauce.

**Nutrition Info:**Calories 190, Fats 10.5g, Carbs 1.8g, Sugar 1g, Proteins 22. Sodium 68mg

## Salmon In Green Sauce

Servings: 4     Cooking Time: 12 Minutes
**Ingredients:**
- 4 (6-ounce) salmon fillets
- 1 avocado, peeled, pitted and chopped
- 1/2 cup fresh basil, chopped
- 3 garlic cloves, chopped
- 1 tablespoon fresh lemon zest, grated finely

**Directions:**
Grease a large piece of foil. In a large bowl, add all ingredients except salmon and water and with a fork, mash completely. Place fillets in the center of foil and top with avocado mixture evenly. Fold the foil around fillets to seal them. Arrange a steamer trivet in the Instant Pot and pour 1/2 cup of water. Place the foil packet on top of trivet. Close the lid and place the pressure valve to "Seal" position. Press "Manual" and cook under "High Pressure" for about minutes. Meanwhile, preheat the oven to broiler. Press "Cancel" and allow a "Natural" release. Open the lid and transfer the salmon fillets onto a broiler pan. Broil for about 3-4 minutes. Serve warm.

**Nutrition Info:**Calories 333, Fats 20.3g, Carbs 5.5g, Sugar 0.4g, Proteins 34.2g, Sodium 79mg

## Blackened Shrimp

Servings: 4     Cooking Time: 5 Minutes
**Ingredients:**
- 1 ½ lbs. shrimp, peel & devein
- 4 lime wedges
- 4 tbsp. cilantro, chopped
- What you'll need from store cupboard:
- 4 cloves garlic, diced
- 1 tbsp. chili powder
- 1 tbsp. paprika
- 1 tbsp. olive oil
- 2 tsp Splenda brown sugar
- 1 tsp cumin
- 1 tsp oregano
- 1 tsp garlic powder
- 1 tsp salt
- ½ tsp pepper

**Directions:**
In a small bowl combine seasonings and Splenda brown sugar.     Heat oil in a skillet over med-high heat. Add shrimp, in a single layer, and cook 1-2 minutes per side. Add seasonings, and cook, stirring, 30 seconds. Serve garnished with cilantro and a lime wedge.
**Nutrition Info:**Calories 252 Total Carbs 7g Net Carbs 6g Protein 39g Fat 7g Sugar 2g Fiber 1g

## Popcorn Shrimp

Servings: 4     Cooking Time: 8 Minutes
**Ingredients:**
- Cooking spray
- ½ cup all-purpose flour
- 2 eggs, beaten
- 2 tablespoons water
- 1 ½ cups panko breadcrumbs
- 1 tablespoon garlic powder
- 1 tablespoon ground cumin
- 1 lb. shrimp, peeled and deveined
- ½ cup ketchup
- 2 tablespoons fresh cilantro, chopped
- 2 tablespoons lime juice
- Salt to taste

**Directions:**
Coat the air fryer basket with cooking spray     Put the flour in a dish.     In the second dish, beat the eggs and water.     In the third dish, mix the breadcrumbs, garlic powder and cumin.     Dip each shrimp in each of the three dishes, first in the dish with flour, then the egg and then breadcrumb mixture.     Place the shrimp in the air fryer basket.     Cook at 360 degrees F for 8 minutes, flipping once halfway through.     Combine the rest of the ingredients as dipping sauce for the shrimp.
**Nutrition Info:**Calories 200 g Fat 25 g Carbohydrates 13.8 g Protein 10 g Cholesterol 21 mg

## Tuna Carbonara

Servings: 4     Cooking Time: 25 Minutes
**Ingredients:**

- ½ lb. tuna fillet, cut in pieces
- 2 eggs
- 4 tbsp. fresh parsley, diced
- What you'll need from store cupboard:
- ½ Homemade Pasta, cook & drain, (chapter 15)
- ½ cup reduced fat parmesan cheese
- 2 cloves garlic, peeled
- 2 tbsp. extra virgin olive oil
- Salt & pepper, to taste

**Directions:**
In a small bowl, beat the eggs, parmesan and a dash of pepper.     Heat the oil in a large skillet over med-high heat. Add garlic and cook until browned. Add the tuna and cook 2-3 minutes, or until tuna is almost cooked through. Discard the garlic.     Add the pasta and reduce heat. Stir in egg mixture and cook, stirring constantly, 2 minutes. If the sauce is too thick, thin with water, a little bit at a time, until it has a creamy texture.     Salt and pepper to taste and serve garnished with parsley.
**Nutrition Info:**Calories 409 Total Carbs 7g Net Carbs 6g Protein 25g Fat 30g Sugar 3g Fiber 1g

## Flavors Cioppino

Servings: 6     Cooking Time: 5 Minutes
**Ingredients:**
- 1 lb codfish, cut into chunks
- 1 1/2 lbs shrimp
- 28 oz can tomatoes, diced
- 1 cup dry white wine
- 1 bay leaf
- 1 tsp cayenne
- 1 tsp oregano
- 1 shallot, chopped
- 1 tsp garlic, minced
- 1 tbsp olive oil
- 1/2 tsp salt

**Directions:**
Add oil into the inner pot of instant pot and set the pot on sauté mode.     Add shallot and garlic and sauté for 2 minutes.     Add wine, bay leaf, cayenne, oregano, and salt and cook for 3 minutes.     Add remaining ingredients and stir well.     Seal pot with a lid and select manual and cook on low for 0 minutes.     Once done, release pressure using quick release. Remove lid. Serve and enjoy.
**Nutrition Info:**Calories 281 Fat 5 g Carbohydrates 10.5 g Sugar 4.9 g Protein 40.7 g Cholesterol 266 mg

## Delicious Shrimp Alfredo

Servings: 4     Cooking Time: 3 Minutes
**Ingredients:**
- 12 shrimp, remove shells
- 1 tbsp garlic, minced
- 1/4 cup parmesan cheese
- 2 cups whole wheat rotini noodles
- 1 cup fish broth
- 15 oz alfredo sauce
- 1 onion, chopped
- Salt

**Directions:**

Add all ingredients except parmesan cheese into the instant pot and stir well. Seal pot with lid and cook on high for 3 minutes. Once done, release pressure using quick release. Remove lid. Stir in cheese and serve.

**Nutrition Info:**Calories 669 Fat 23.1 g Carbohydrates 76 g Sugar 2.4 g Protein 37.8 g Cholesterol 190 mg

## Salmon & Asparagus

Servings: 2    Cooking Time: 10 Minutes
**Ingredients:**
- 2 salmon fillets
- 8 spears asparagus, trimmed
- 2 tablespoons balsamic vinegar
- 1 teaspoon olive oil
- 1 teaspoon dried dill
- Salt and pepper to taste

**Directions:**
Preheat your oven to 325 degrees F. Dry salmon with paper towels. Arrange the asparagus around the salmon fillets on a baking pan. In a bowl, mix the rest of the ingredients. Pour mixture over the salmon and vegetables. Bake in the oven for 10 minutes or until the fish is fully cooked.

**Nutrition Info:**Calories 150 g Fat 22 g Carbohydrates 13.6 g Protein 7 g Cholesterol 20 mg

## Tuna Sweet Corn Casserole

Servings: 2    Cooking Time: 35 Minutes
**Ingredients:**
- 3 small tins of tuna
- 0.5lb sweet corn kernels
- 1lb chopped vegetables
- 1 cup low sodium vegetable broth
- 2tbsp spicy seasoning

**Directions:**
Mix all the ingredients in your Instant Pot. Cook on Stew for 35 minutes. Release the pressure naturally.

**Nutrition Info:**Calories: 300;Carbs: 6 ;Sugar: 1 ;Fat: 9 ;Protein: ;GL: 2

## Tortilla Chip With Black Bean Salad

Servings: 4    Cooking Time: 20 Minutes
**Ingredients:**
- 4 oz. white fish fillets and tortilla chips
- 1/3 cup frozen egg, thawed
- ¼ red onion, chopped
- ¼ teaspoon cumin, ground
- ½ cup cherry tomatoes, halved
- What you will need from the store cupboard:
- 2 teaspoons olive oil
- 1 tablespoon lemon juice
- ¼ teaspoon cayenne pepper
- ½ cup green bell pepper, chopped
- ¼ teaspoon salt
- Cooking spray

**Directions:**
Preheat your oven to 350 ºF. Use a foil to line your baking sheet. Apply cooking spray on the foil. Combine the cayenne pepper and tortilla chips in your food processor. Cover till it is crushed fine. Keep in a dish. Use paper towels to pat dry. Pour egg into a second dish. Dip your fish into this and then in your tortilla chips. Now keep the fish on the baking sheet. Coat it with cooking spray lightly. Bake for 8 minutes. The fish must flake easily with a fork. In the meantime, for the salad, bring together the tomatoes, onion, lemon juice, bell pepper, cumin, salt, and oil in your bowl. Place fish on top of the salad. Sprinkle some cheese on top.

**Nutrition Info:**Calories 361, Carbohydrates 35g, Fiber 8g, Sugar 0.3g, Cholesterol 46mg, Total Fat 11g, Protein 28g

## Crunchy Lemon Shrimp

Servings: 4    Cooking Time: 10 Minutes,
**Ingredients:**
- 1 lb. raw shrimp, peeled and deveined
- 2 tbsp. Italian parsley, roughly chopped
- 2 tbsp. lemon juice, divided
- What you'll need from store cupboard:
- ⅔ cup panko bread crumbs
- 2½ tbsp. olive oil, divided
- Salt and pepper, to taste

**Directions:**
Heat oven to 400 degrees. Place the shrimp evenly in a baking dish and sprinkle with salt and pepper. Drizzle on 1 tablespoon lemon juice and 1 tablespoon of olive oil. Set aside. In a medium bowl, combine parsley, remaining lemon juice, bread crumbs, remaining olive oil, and ¼ tsp each of salt and pepper. Layer the panko mixture evenly on top of the shrimp. Bake 8-10 minutes or until shrimp are cooked through and the panko is golden brown.

**Nutrition Info:**Calories 283 Total Carbs 15g Net Carbs 14g Protein 28g Fat 12g Sugar 1g Fiber 1g

## Fish Amandine

Servings: 4    Cooking Time: 15 Minutes
**Ingredients:**
- 4 oz. frozen or fresh tilapia, halibut or trout fillets (skinless, 1-inch size)
- 1/8 teaspoon red pepper, crushed
- ¼ cup almonds, chopped
- ½ cup bread crumbs
- 2 tablespoons parsley, chopped
- What you will need from the store cupboard:
- ½ teaspoon dry mustard
- ¼ cup buttermilk
- 1 tablespoon melted butter
- 2 tablespoons Parmesan cheese, grated
- ¼ teaspoon salt

**Directions:**
Preheat your oven to 350 ºF and grease the baking pan. Keep it aside. Rinse the fish. Use paper towels to pat dry. Now pour the buttermilk into a dish. Take another dish and bring together the parsley, bread crumbs, salt, and dry mustard. Place fish into the buttermilk. Then into your crumb mix. Now keep the coated fish in the baking pan. Sprinkle Parmesan cheese and almonds on the fish. Drizzle melted butter.

Also, sprinkle the crushed red pepper.    Bake for 4-6 minutes.
**Nutrition Info:**Calories 209, Carbohydrates 7g, Fiber 1g, Sugar 1g, Cholesterol 67mg, Total Fat 9g, Protein 26g

## Shrimp & Veggies Curry

Servings: 6      Cooking Time: 20 Minutes
**Ingredients:**
- 2 teaspoons olive oil
- 1½ medium white onions, sliced
- 2 medium green bell peppers, seeded and sliced
- 3 medium carrots, peeled and sliced thinly
- 3 garlic cloves, chopped finely
- 1 tablespoon fresh ginger, chopped finely
- 2½ teaspoons curry powder
- 1½ pounds shrimp, peeled and deveined
- 1 cup filtered water
- 2 tablespoons fresh lime juice
- Salt and ground black pepper, as required
- 2 tablespoons fresh cilantro, chopped

**Directions:**
In a large skillet, heat oil over medium-high heat and sauté the onion for about 4-5 minutes.    Add the bell peppers and carrot and sauté for about 3-4 minutes. Add the garlic, ginger and curry powder and sauté for about 1 minute.    Add the shrimp and sauté for about 1 minute.    Stir in the water and cook for about 4-6 minutes, stirring occasionally.    Stir in lime juice and remove from heat.    Serve hot with the garnishing of cilantro.    Meal Prep Tip: Transfer the curry into a large bowl and set aside to cool. Divide the curry into 6 containers evenly. Cover the containers and refrigerate for 1-2 days. Reheat in the microwave before serving.
**Nutrition Info:**Calories 193 Total Fat 3.8 g Saturated Fat 0.9 g Cholesterol 239 mg Total Carbs 12 g Sugar 4.7 g Fiber 2.3 g Sodium 328 mg Potassium 437 mg Protein 27.1 g

## Coconut Clam Chowder

Servings: 6      Cooking Time: 7 Minutes
**Ingredients:**
- 6 oz clams, chopped
- 1 cup heavy cream
- 1/4 onion, sliced
- 1 cup celery, chopped
- 1 lb cauliflower, chopped
- 1 cup fish broth
- 1 bay leaf
- 2 cups of coconut milk
- Salt

**Directions:**
Add all ingredients except clams and heavy cream and stir well.    Seal pot with lid and cook on high for 5 minutes.    Once done, release pressure using quick release. Remove lid.    Add heavy cream and clams and stir well and cook on sauté mode for 2 minutes.    Stir well and serve.
**Nutrition Info:**Calories 301 Fat 27.2 g Carbohydrates 13.6 g Sugar 6 g Protein 4.9 g Cholesterol 33 mg

## Lemon Pepper Salmon

Servings: 4      Cooking Time: 10 Minutes
**Ingredients:**
- 3 tbsps. ghee or avocado oil
- 1 lb. skin-on salmon filet
- 1 julienned red bell pepper
- 1 julienned green zucchini
- 1 julienned carrot
- ¾ cup water
- A few sprigs of parsley, tarragon, dill, basil or a combination
- 1/2 sliced lemon
- 1/2 tsp. black pepper
- ¼ tsp. sea salt

**Directions:**
Add the water and the herbs into the bottom of the Instant Pot and put in a wire steamer rack making sure the handles extend upwards.    Place the salmon filet onto the wire rack, with the skin side facing down. Drizzle the salmon with ghee, season with black pepper and salt, and top with the lemon slices.    Close and seal the Instant Pot, making sure the vent is turned to "Sealing".    Select the "Steam" setting and cook for 3 minutes.    While the salmon cooks, julienne the vegetables, and set aside.    Once done, quick release the pressure, and then press the "Keep Warm/Cancel" button.    Uncover and wearing oven mitts, carefully remove the steamer rack with the salmon.    Remove the herbs and discard them.    Add the vegetables to the pot and put the lid back on.    Select the "Sauté" function and cook for 1-2 minutes.    Serve the vegetables with salmon and add the remaining fat to the pot.    Pour a little of the sauce over the fish and vegetables if desired.
**Nutrition Info:**Calories 296, Carbs 8g, Fat 15 g, Protein 31 g, Potassium (K) 1084 mg, Sodium (Na) 284 mg

## Tomato Olive Fish Fillets

Servings: 4      Cooking Time: 8 Minutes
**Ingredients:**
- 2 lbs halibut fish fillets
- 2 oregano sprigs
- 2 rosemary sprigs
- 2 tbsp fresh lime juice
- 1 cup olives, pitted
- 28 oz can tomatoes, diced
- 1 tbsp garlic, minced
- 1 onion, chopped
- 2 tbsp olive oil

**Directions:**
Add oil into the inner pot of instant pot and set the pot on sauté mode.    Add onion and sauté for 3 minutes. Add garlic and sauté for a minute.    Add lime juice, olives, herb sprigs, and tomatoes and stir well.    Seal pot with lid and cook on high for 3 minutes.    Once done, release pressure using quick release. Remove lid. Add fish fillets and seal pot again with lid and cook on high for 2 minutes.    Once done, release pressure using quick release. Remove lid.    Serve and enjoy.
**Nutrition Info:**Calories 333 Fat 19.1 g Carbohydrates 31.8 g Sugar 8.4 g Protein 13.4 g Cholesterol 5 mg

## Almond Crusted Baked Chili Mahi Mahi

Servings: 4    Cooking Time: 15 Minutes

**Ingredients:**
- 4 mahi mahi fillets
- 1 lime
- 2 teaspoons olive oil
- Salt and pepper to taste
- ½ cup almonds
- ¼ teaspoon paprika
- ¼ teaspoon onion powder
- ¾ teaspoon chili powder
- ½ cup red bell pepper, chopped
- ¼ cup onion, chopped
- ¼ cup fresh cilantro, chopped

**Directions:**
Preheat your oven to 325 degrees F.    Line your baking pan with parchment paper.    Squeeze juice from the lime.    Grate zest from the peel.    Put juice and zest in a bowl.    Add the oil, salt and pepper.    In another bowl, add the almonds, paprika, onion powder and chili powder.    Put the almond mixture in a food processor. Pulse until powdery.    Dip each fillet in the oil mixture. Dredge with the almond and chili mixture.    Arrange on a single layer in the oven.    Bake for 12 to 15 minutes or until fully cooked.    Serve with red bell pepper, onion and cilantro.

**Nutrition Info:** Calories 322 Total Fat 12 g Saturated Fat 2 g Cholesterol 83 mg Sodium 328 mg Total Carbohydrate 28 g Dietary Fiber 4 g Total Sugars 10 g Protein 28 g Potassium 829 mg

## Shrimp Lemon Kebab

Servings: 5    Cooking Time: 4 Minutes

**Ingredients:**
- 1 ½ lb. shrimp, peeled and deveined but with tails intact
- ⅓ cup olive oil
- ¼ cup lemon juice
- 2 teaspoons lemon zest
- 1 tablespoon fresh parsley, chopped
- 8 cherry tomatoes, quartered
- 2 scallions, sliced

**Directions:**
Mix the olive oil, lemon juice, lemon zest and parsley in a bowl.    Marinate the shrimp in this mixture for 15 minutes.    Thread each shrimp into the skewers. Grill for 4 to 5 minutes, turning once halfway through. Serve with tomatoes and scallions.

**Nutrition Info:** Calories 180 g Fat 20 g Carbohydrates 15 g Protein 11 g Cholesterol 26 mg

## Turkish Tuna With Bulgur And Chickpea Salad

Servings: 4    Cooking Time: 20 Minutes

**Ingredients:**
- 16 oz. tuna, 4 steaks
- ½ cup bulgur
- 12 oz. chickpeas
- 4 teaspoons lemon zest, grated
- ¼ cup Italian parsley, chopped
- What you will need from the store cupboard:
- ¼ cup extra-virgin olive oil
- ¼ teaspoon ground pepper
- ½ teaspoon salt

**Directions:**
Boil water and keep the bulgur in your bowl.    Add 2 inches of the water.    Mix your bulgur with 1 tablespoon of oil, pepper, salt, and the lemon zest.    Add the chickpeas and parsley.    Stir well to combine.    Now heat the remaining oil in your skillet over medium heat. Add the tuna. Sear both sides until they become brown. The tuna should flake easily with your fork. Transfer to a plate.    In the meantime, bring together ¼ teaspoon salt and the remaining lemon zest in a bowl.    Transfer your tuna fish to a serving platter.    Sprinkle lemon zest and serve with the bulgur.

**Nutrition Info:** Calories 459, Carbohydrates 43g, Fiber 8g, Sugar 0.2g, Cholesterol 44mg, Total Fat 16g, Protein 36g

## Cajun Flounder & Tomatoes

Servings: 4    Cooking Time: 15 Minutes

**Ingredients:**
- 4 flounder fillets
- 2 ½ cups tomatoes, diced
- ¾ cup onion, diced
- ¾ cup green bell pepper, diced
- What you'll need from store cupboard:
- 2 cloves garlic, diced fine
- 1 tbsp. Cajun seasoning
- 1 tsp olive oil

**Directions:**
Heat oil in a large skillet over med-high heat. Add onion and garlic and cook 2 minutes, or until soft. Add tomatoes, peppers and spices, and cook 2-3 minutes until tomatoes soften.    Lay fish over top. Cover, reduce heat to medium and cook, 5-8 minutes, or until fish flakes easily with a fork. Transfer fish to serving plates and top with sauce.

**Nutrition Info:** Calories 194 Total Carbs 8g Net Carbs 6g Protein 32g Fat 3g Sugar 5g Fiber 2g

## Lemon Sole

Servings: 2    Cooking Time: 5 Minutes

**Ingredients:**
- 1lb sole fillets, boned and skinned
- 1 cup low sodium fish broth
- 2 shredded sweet onions
- juice of half a lemon
- 2tbsp dried cilantro

**Directions:**
Mix all the ingredients in your Instant Pot.    Cook on Stew for 5 minutes.    Release the pressure naturally.

**Nutrition Info:** Calories 230; Carbs Sugar 1; Fat 6; Protein 46; GL 1

## Trout Bake

Servings: 2    Cooking Time: 35 Minutes

**Ingredients:**
- 1lb trout fillets, boneless

- 1lb chopped winter vegetables
- 1 cup low sodium fish broth
- 1tbsp mixed herbs
- sea salt as desired

**Directions:**
Mix all the ingredients except the broth in a foil pouch. Place the pouch in the steamer basket your Instant Pot. Pour the broth into the Instant Pot.    Cook on Steam for 35 minutes.    Release the pressure naturally.
**Nutrition Info:**Calories 310; Carbs 14; Sugar 2; Fat 12; Protein 40; GL 5

## Garlic Shrimp & Spinach

Servings: 4    Cooking Time: 10 Minutes
**Ingredients:**
- 3 tablespoons olive oil, divided
- 6 clove garlic, sliced and divided
- 1 lb. spinach
- Salt to taste
- 1 tablespoons lemon juice
- 1 lb. shrimp, peeled and deveined
- ¼ teaspoon red pepper, crushed
- 1 tablespoon parsley, chopped
- 1 teaspoon lemon zest

**Directions:**
Pour 1 tablespoon olive oil in a pot over medium heat. Cook the garlic for 1 minute.    Add the spinach and season with salt.    Cook for 3 minutes.    Stir in lemon juice.    Transfer to a bowl.    Pour the remaining oil. Add the shrimp.    Season with salt and add red pepper. Cook for 5 minutes.    Sprinkle parsley and lemon zest over the shrimp before serving.
**Nutrition Info:**Calories 226 Total Fat 12 g Saturated Fat 2 g Cholesterol 183 mg Sodium 444 mg Total Carbohydrate 6 g Dietary Fiber 3 g Total Sugars 1 g Protein 26 g Potassium 963 mg

## Salmon With Bell Peppers

Servings: 6    Cooking Time: 20 Minutes
**Ingredients:**
- 6 (3-ounce) salmon fillets
- Pinch of salt
- Ground black pepper, as required
- 1 yellow bell pepper, seeded and cubed
- 1 red bell pepper, seeded and cubed
- 4 plum tomatoes, cubed
- 1 small onion, sliced thinly
- ½ cup fresh parsley, chopped
- ¼ cup olive oil
- 2 tablespoons fresh lemon juice

**Directions:**
Preheat the oven to 400 degrees F.    Season each salmon fillet with salt and black pepper lightly.    In a bowl, mix together the bell peppers, tomato and onion. Arrange 6 foil pieces onto a smooth surface.    Place 1 salmon fillet over each foil paper and sprinkle with salt and black pepper.    Place veggie mixture over each fillet evenly and top with parsley and capers evenly.    Drizzle with oil and lemon juice.    Fold each foil around salmon mixture to seal it.    Arrange the foil packets onto a large baking sheet in a single layer.    Bake for about 20

minutes.    Serve hot.    Meal Prep Tip: Transfer the salmon mixture into a large bowl and set aside to cool. Divide the salmon mixture into 6 containers evenly. Cover the containers and refrigerate for 1 day. Reheat in the microwave before serving.
**Nutrition Info:**Calories 220 Total Fat 14 g Saturated Fat 2 g Cholesterol 38 mg Total Carbs 7.7 g Sugar 4.8 g Fiber 2 g Sodium 74 mg Potassium 647 mg Protein 17.9 g

## Tarragon Scallops

Servings: 4    Cooking Time: 15 Minutes
**Ingredients:**
- 1 cup water
- 1 lb. asparagus spears, trimmed
- 2 lemons
- 1 ¼ lb. scallops
- Salt and pepper to taste
- 1 tablespoon olive oil
- 1 tablespoon fresh tarragon, chopped

**Directions:**
Pour water into a pot.    Bring to a boil.    Add asparagus spears.    Cover and cook for 5 minutes. Drain and transfer to a plate.    Slice one lemon into wedges.    Squeeze juice and shred zest from the remaining lemon.    Season the scallops with salt and pepper.    Put a pan over medium heat.    Add oil to the pan.    Cook the scallops until golden brown. Transfer to the same plate, putting scallops beside the asparagus.    Add lemon zest, juice and tarragon to the pan.    Cook for 1 minute.    Drizzle tarragon sauce over the scallops and asparagus.
**Nutrition Info:**Calories 253 Total Fat 12 g Saturated Fat 2 g Cholesterol 47 mg Sodium 436 mg Total Carbohydrate 14 g Dietary Fiber 5 g Total Sugars 3 g Protein 27 g Potassium 773 mg

## Salmon Curry

Servings: 6    Cooking Time: 30 Minutes
**Ingredients:**
- 6 (4-ounce) salmon fillets
- 1 teaspoon ground turmeric, divided
- Salt, as required
- 3 tablespoon olive oil, divided
- 1 yellow onion, chopped finely
- 1 teaspoon garlic paste
- 1 teaspoon fresh ginger paste
- 3-4 green chilies, halved
- 1 teaspoon red chili powder
- ½ teaspoon ground cumin
- ½ teaspoon ground cinnamon
- ¾ cup fat-free plain Greek yogurt, whipped
- ¾ cup filtered water
- 3 tablespoon fresh cilantro, chopped

**Directions:**
Season each salmon fillet with ½ teaspoon of the turmeric and salt.    In a large skillet, melt 1 tablespoon of the butter over medium heat and cook the salmon fillets for about 2 minutes per side.    Transfer the salmon onto a plate.    In the same skillet, melt the remaining butter over medium heat and sauté the onion

for about 4-5 minutes. Add the garlic paste, ginger paste, green chilies, remaining turmeric and spices and sauté for about 1 minute. Now, reduce the heat to medium-low. Slowly, add the yogurt and water, stirring continuously until smooth. Cover the skillet and simmer for about 10-15 minutes or until desired doneness of the sauce. Carefully, add the salmon fillets and simmer for about 5 minutes. Serve hot with the garnishing of cilantro. Meal Prep Tip: Transfer the curry into a large bowl and set aside to cool. Divide the curry into 6 containers evenly. Cover the containers and refrigerate for 1-2 days. Reheat in the microwave before serving.

**Nutrition Info:**Calories 242 Total Fat 14.3 g Saturated Fat 2 g Cholesterol 51 mg Total Carbs 4.1 g Sugar 2 g Fiber 0.8 g Sodium 98 mg Potassium 493 mg Protein 25.4 g

## Halibut With Spicy Apricot Sauce

Servings: 4      Cooking Time: 17 Minutes
**Ingredients:**
- 4 fresh apricots, pitted
- ⅓ cup apricot preserves
- ½ cup apricot nectar
- ½ teaspoon dried oregano
- 3 tablespoons scallion, sliced
- 1 teaspoon hot pepper sauce
- Salt to taste
- 4 halibut steaks
- 1 tablespoon olive oil

**Directions:**
Put the apricots, preserves, nectar, oregano, scallion, hot pepper sauce and salt in a saucepan. Bring to a boil and then simmer for 8 minutes. Set aside. Brush the halibut steaks with olive oil. Grill for 7 to 9 minutes or until fish is flaky. Brush one tablespoon of the sauce on both sides of the fish. Serve with the reserved sauce.

**Nutrition Info:**Calories 304 Total Fat 8 g Saturated Fat 1 g Cholesterol 73 mg Sodium 260 mg Total Carbohydrate 27 g Dietary Fiber 2 g Total Sugars 16 g Protein 29 g Potassium 637 mg

## Easy Salmon Stew

Servings: 6      Cooking Time: 8 Minutes
**Ingredients:**
- 2 lbs salmon fillet, cubed
- 1 onion, chopped
- 2 cups fish broth
- 1 tbsp olive oil
- Pepper
- salt

**Directions:**
Add oil into the inner pot of instant pot and set the pot on sauté mode. Add onion and sauté for 2 minutes. Add remaining ingredients and stir well. Seal pot with lid and cook on high for 6 minutes. Once done, release pressure using quick release. Remove lid. Stir and serve.

**Nutrition Info:**Calories 243 Fat 12.6 g Carbohydrates 0.8 g Sugar 0.3 g Protein 31 g Cholesterol 78 mg

## Cilantro Lime Grilled Shrimp

Servings: 6      Cooking Time: 5 Minutes,
**Ingredients:**
- 1 ½ lbs. large shrimp raw, peeled, deveined with tails on
- Juice and zest of 1 lime
- 2 tbsp. fresh cilantro chopped
- What you'll need from store cupboard:
- ¼ cup olive oil
- 2 cloves garlic, diced fine
- 1 tsp smoked paprika
- ¼ tsp cumin
- ½ teaspoon salt
- ¼ tsp cayenne pepper

**Directions:**
Place the shrimp in a large Ziploc bag. Mix remaining Ingredients in a small bowl and pour over shrimp. Let marinate 20-30 minutes. Heat up the grill. Skewer the shrimp and cook 2-3 minutes, per side, just until they turn pick. Be careful not to overcook them. Serve garnished with cilantro.

**Nutrition Info:**Calories 317 Total Carbs 4g Protein 39g Fat 15g Sugar 0g Fiber 0g

## Cajun Catfish

Servings: 4      Cooking Time: 15 Minutes
**Ingredients:**
- 4 (8 oz.) catfish fillets
- What you'll need from store cupboard:
- 2 tbsp. olive oil
- 2 tsp garlic salt
- 2 tsp thyme
- 2 tsp paprika
- ½ tsp cayenne pepper
- ½ tsp red hot sauce
- ¼ tsp black pepper
- Nonstick cooking spray

**Directions:**
Heat oven to 450 degrees. Spray a 9x13-inch baking dish with cooking spray. In a small bowl whisk together everything but catfish. Brush both sides of fillets, using all the spice mix. Bake 10-13 minutes or until fish flakes easily with a fork. Serve.

**Nutrition Info:**Calories 366 Total Carbs 0g Protein 35g Fat 24g Sugar 0g Fiber 0g

## Halibut With Spicy Apricot Sauce

Servings: 4      Cooking Time: 17 Minutes
**Ingredients:**
- 4 fresh apricots, pitted
- ⅓ cup apricot preserves
- ½ cup apricot nectar
- ½ teaspoon dried oregano
- 3 tablespoons scallion, sliced
- 1 teaspoon hot pepper sauce
- Salt to taste
- 4 halibut steaks
- 1 tablespoon olive oil

**Directions:**

Put the apricots, preserves, nectar, oregano, scallion, hot pepper sauce and salt in a saucepan. Bring to a boil and then simmer for 8 minutes. Set aside. Brush the halibut steaks with olive oil. Grill for 7 to 9 minutes or until fish is flaky. Brush one tablespoon of the sauce on both sides of the fish. Serve with the reserved sauce. Bake in the oven for 10 minutes or until the fish is fully cooked.

**Nutrition Info:**Calories 150 g Fat 22 g Carbohydrates 13.6 g Protein 7 g Cholesterol 20 mg

## Mixed Chowder

Servings: 2    Cooking Time: 35 Minutes
**Ingredients:**
- 1lb fish stew mix
- 2 cups white sauce
- 3tbsp old bay seasoning

**Directions:**
Mix all the ingredients in your Instant Pot. Cook on Stew for 35 minutes. Release the pressure naturally.

**Nutrition Info:**Calories 320; Carbs 9; Sugar 2; Fat 16; Protein GL 4

## Shrimp With Zucchini

Servings: 4    Cooking Time: 8 Minutes
**Ingredients:**
- 3 tablespoons olive oil
- 1 pound medium shrimp, peeled and deveined
- 1 shallot, minced
- 4 garlic cloves, minced
- ¼ teaspoon red pepper flakes, crushed
- Salt and ground black pepper, as required
- ¼ cup low-sodium chicken broth
- 2 tablespoons fresh lemon juice
- 1 teaspoon fresh lemon zest, grated finely
- ½ pound zucchini, spiralized with Blade C

**Directions:**
In a large skillet, heat the oil and butter over medium-high heat and cook the shrimp, shallot, garlic, red pepper flakes, salt and black pepper for about 2 minutes, stirring occasionally. Stir in the broth, lemon juice and lemon zest and bring to a gentle boil. Stir in zucchini noodles and cook for about 1-2 minutes. Serve hot. Meal Prep Tip: Transfer the shrimp mixture into a large bowl and set aside to cool. Divide the shrimp mixture into 4 containers. Cover the containers and refrigerate for about 1-2 days. Reheat in microwave before serving.

**Nutrition Info:**Calories 245 Total Fat 12.6 g Saturated Fat 2.2 g Cholesterol 239 mg Total Carbs 5.8 g Sugar 1.2 g Fiber 08 g Sodium 289 mg Potassium 381 mg Protein 27 g

## Braised Shrimp

Servings: 4    Cooking Time: 4 Minutes
**Ingredients:**
- 1 pound frozen large shrimp, peeled and deveined
- 2 shallots, chopped
- ¾ cup low-sodium chicken broth
- 2 tablespoons fresh lemon juice
- 2 tablespoons olive oil

- 1 tablespoon garlic, crushed
- Ground black pepper, as required

**Directions:**
In the Instant Pot, place oil and press "Sauté". Now add the shallots and cook for about 2 minutes. Add the garlic and cook for about 1 minute. Press "Cancel" and stir in the shrimp, broth, lemon juice and black pepper. Close the lid and place the pressure valve to "Seal" position. Press "Manual" and cook under "High Pressure" for about 1 minute. Press "Cancel" and carefully allow a "Quick" release. Open the lid and serve hot.

**Nutrition Info:**Calories 209, Fats 9g, Carbs 4.3g, Sugar 0.2g, Proteins 26.6g, Sodium 293mg

## Salmon Soup

Servings: 4    Cooking Time: 20 Minutes
**Ingredients:**
- 1 tablespoon olive oil
- 1 yellow onion, chopped
- 1 garlic clove, minced
- 4 cups low-sodium chicken broth
- 1 pound boneless salmon, cubed
- 2 tablespoon fresh cilantro, chopped
- Ground black pepper, as required
- 1 tablespoon fresh lime juice

**Directions:**
In a large pan heat the oil over medium heat and sauté the onion for about 5 minutes. Add the garlic and sauté for about 1 minute. Stir in the broth and bring to a boil over high heat. Now, reduce the heat to low and simmer for about 10 minutes. Add the salmon, and soy sauce and cook for about 3-4 minutes. Stir in black pepper, lime juice, and cilantro and serve hot. Meal Prep Tip: Transfer the soup into a large bowl and set aside to cool. Divide the soup into 4 containers evenly. Cover the containers and refrigerate for 1-2 days. Reheat in the microwave before serving.

**Nutrition Info:**Calories 208 Total Fat 10.5 g Saturated Fat 1.5 g Cholesterol 50 mg Total Carbs 3.9 g Sugar 1.2 g Fiber 0.6 g Sodium 121 mg Potassium 331 mg Protein 24.4 g

## Salmon With Pineapple-cilantro Salsa

Servings: 4    Cooking Time: 15 Minutes
**Ingredients:**
- 1 lb. salmon fillets, skinless, 1 inch thick
- 2 tablespoons parsley or cilantro, chopped
- 2 cups pineapple, chopped
- ¼ cup red onion, chopped
- ½ cup green or red bell pepper, chopped
- What you will need from the store cupboard:
- ¼ teaspoon salt
- ½ teaspoon chili powder
- 3 tablespoons lime juice
- Lime wedges, optional
- Pinch of cayenne pepper

**Directions:**
Rinse the fish. Use paper towels to pat dry. For the salsa, bring together the bell pepper, pineapple, lime juice, red onion, and a tablespoon of parsley or cilantro

in a bowl. Keep this aside.    Now combine the lime juice, salt, and the remaining parsley or cilantro.    Brush this on both sides of your fish.    Keep fish on your grill and grill for 8 minutes. Turn once.    Cut your fish into 4 serving sizes. Apply salsa on top.    You can serve with lettuce and lime wedges.

**Nutrition Info:** Calories 257, Carbohydrates 13g, Fiber 2g, Sugar 1g, Cholesterol 66mg, Total Fat 12g, Protein 23g

### Italian Tuna Pasta

Servings: 6    Cooking Time: 5 Minutes

**Ingredients:**
- 15 oz whole wheat pasta
- 2 tbsp capers
- 3 oz tuna
- 2 cups can tomatoes, crushed
- 2 anchovies
- 1 tsp garlic, minced
- 1 tbsp olive oil
- Salt

**Directions:**
Add oil into the inner pot of instant pot and set the pot on sauté mode.    Add anchovies and garlic and sauté for 1 minute.    Add remaining ingredients and stir well. Pour enough water into the pot to cover the pasta. Seal pot with a lid and select manual and cook on low for 4 minutes.    Once done, release pressure using quick release. Remove lid.    Stir and serve.

**Nutrition Info:** Calories 339 Fat 6 g Carbohydrates 56.5 g Sugar 5.2 g Protein 15.2 g Cholesterol 10 mg

### Baked Salmon With Garlic Parmesan Topping

Servings: 4    Cooking Time: 20 Minutes,

**Ingredients:**
- 1 lb. wild caught salmon filets
- 2 tbsp. margarine
- What you'll need from store cupboard:
- ¼ cup reduced fat parmesan cheese, grated
- ¼ cup light mayonnaise
- 2-3 cloves garlic, diced
- 2 tbsp. parsley
- Salt and pepper

**Directions:**
Heat oven to 350 and line a baking pan with parchment paper.    Place salmon on pan and season with salt and pepper.    In a medium skillet, over medium heat, melt butter. Add garlic and cook, stirring 1 minute.    Reduce heat to low and add remaining Ingredients. Stir until everything is melted and combined.    Spread evenly over salmon and bake 15 minutes for thawed fish or 20 for frozen. Salmon is done when it flakes easily with a fork. Serve.

**Nutrition Info:** Calories 408 Total Carbs 4g Protein 41g Fat 24g Sugar 1g Fiber 0g

# Vegetable Recipes

## Cucumber Salad With Pesto

Servings: 4    Cooking Time: 0 Minute

**Ingredients:**
- 1 cup fresh basil leaves, chopped
- 2 cloves garlic
- 2 tablespoons walnuts
- 1 teaspoon Parmesan cheese
- 1 tablespoon olive oil
- 2 cucumbers, sliced into rounds
- Salt and pepper to taste

**Directions:**
Put the basil, garlic, walnuts, Parmesan cheese and olive oil in a food processor. Pulse until smooth. Season the cucumbers with salt and pepper. Spread pesto on top of each cucumber round.

**Nutrition Info:** Calories 80 Total Fat 6g Saturated Fat 0.7g Cholesterol 0mg Sodium 4mg Total Carbohydrate 6.5g Dietary Fiber 1.2g Total Sugars 2.6g Protein 2.2g Potassium 266mg

## Easy Brussels Sprouts Hash

Servings: 4    Cooking Time: 10 Minutes

**Ingredients:**
- 3 tablespoons extra-virgin olive oil
- 1 onion, finely chopped
- 1 pound Brussels sprouts, bottoms trimmed off, shredded (see tip)
- ½ teaspoon caraway seeds
- ½ teaspoon sea salt
- ⅛ teaspoon freshly ground black pepper
- ¼ cup red wine vinegar
- 1 tablespoon Dijon mustard
- 1 tablespoon honey
- 3 garlic cloves, minced

**Directions:**
In a large skillet over medium-high heat, heat the olive oil until it shimmers. Add the onion, Brussels sprouts, caraway seeds, sea salt, and pepper. Cook for 7 to 10 minutes, stirring occasionally, until the Brussels sprouts begin to brown. While the Brussels sprouts cook, whisk the vinegar, mustard, and honey in a small bowl and set aside. Add the garlic to the skillet and cook for 30 seconds, stirring constantly. Add the vinegar mixture to the skillet. Cook for about 5 minutes, stirring, until the liquid reduces by half.

**Nutrition Info:** Calories: 176; Protein: 11g; Total Carbohydrates: 19g; Sugars: 8g; Fiber: 5g; Total Fat: 11g; Saturated Fat: 1g; Cholesterol: 0mg; Sodium: 309mg

## Vegetable And Bean Stew

Servings: 6    Cooking Time: 20 Minutes

**Ingredients:**
- 1 lb. potatoes, cut into small 1 inch chunks
- 2 parsnips, 1-inch chunks
- 2 carrots, 1-inch chunks
- 19 oz. pinto beans, drained and rinsed
- 1 acorn squash
- What you will need from the store cupboard:
- 2 teaspoons olive oil
- 1 cup apple cider
- 1 cup vegetable broth, low-sodium
- Salt and pepper to taste

**Directions:**
Preheat your oven to 350 °F. Divide the squash. Remove the seeds. Cut the flesh into 4 cm chunks and peel the skin. Put them in a bowl and also the carrots, potatoes, and parsnips. Drizzle olive oil. Toss well to coat. Now stir the garlic in. Season with pepper and salt lightly. Keep the rosemary sprigs in your roasting pan. Spread vegetables in a single layer on top. Roast to brown lightly. Turn once. Take out from the oven. Stir the cider, broth and pinto beans in. Use foil to cover your pan tightly. Cook until your vegetables have become tender. Garnish with rosemary sprigs.

**Nutrition Info:** Calories 278, Fat 3g, Protein 8g, Carbohydrates 58g, Fiber 11g, Cholesterol 0mg, Sugar 0.6g

## Grilled Zucchini With Tomato Relish

Servings: 4    Cooking Time: 10 Minutes

**Ingredients:**
- 1 lb. zucchini, sliced in half
- 1 tablespoon olive oil
- Salt and pepper to taste
- 1 teaspoon red wine vinegar
- 1 tablespoon mint, chopped
- 1 cup tomatoes, chopped

**Directions:**
Preheat your grill. Brush both sides of zucchini with oil and season with salt and pepper. Grill for 3 to 4 minutes per side. In a bowl, mix the rest of the ingredients with the remaining oil. Season with salt and pepper. Spread tomato relish on top of the grilled zucchini before serving.

**Nutrition Info:** Calories 71 Total Fat 5 g Saturated Fat 1 g Cholesterol 0 mg Sodium 157 mg Total Carbohydrate 6 g Dietary Fiber 2 g Total Sugars 4 g Protein 2 g Potassium 413 mg

## Carrot Soup With Tempeh

Servings: 6    Cooking Time: 45 Minutes

**Ingredients:**
- ¼ cup olive oil, divided
- 1 large yellow onion, chopped
- Salt, to taste
- 2 pounds' carrots, peeled, and cut into ½-inch rounds
- 2 tablespoons fresh dill, chopped
- 4½ cups homemade vegetable broth
- 12 ounces' tempeh, cut into ½-inch cubes
- ¼ cup tomato paste
- 1 teaspoon fresh lemon juice

**Directions:**

In a large soup pan, heat 2 tablespoons of the oil over medium heat and cook the onion with salt for about 6–8 minutes, stirring frequently. Add the carrots and stir to combine. Lower the heat to low and cook, covered for about 5 minutes, stirring frequently. Add in the broth and bring to a boil over high heat. Lower the heat to a low and simmer, covered for about 30 minutes. Meanwhile, in a skillet, heat the remaining oil over medium-high heat and cook the tempeh for about 3–5 minutes. Stir in the dill and cook for about 1 minute. Remove from the heat. Remove the pan of soup from heat and stir in tomato paste and lemon juice. With an immersion blender, blend the soup until smooth and creamy. Serve the soup hot with the topping of tempeh.

**Nutrition Info:** Calories 294 Total Fat 15.7 g Saturated Fat 2.8 g Cholesterol 0 mg Sodium 723 mg Total Carbs 25.9 g Fiber 4.9 g Sugar 10.4 g Protein 16.4 g

## Beet Soup

Servings: 2    Cooking Time: 5 Minutes

**Ingredients:**
- 2 cups coconut yogurt
- 4 teaspoons fresh lemon juice
- 2 cups beets, trimmed, peeled, and chopped
- 2 tablespoons fresh dill
- Salt, to taste
- 1 tablespoon pumpkin seeds
- 2 tablespoons coconut cream
- 1 tablespoon fresh chives, minced

**Directions:**
In a high-speed blender, add all ingredients and pulse until smooth. Transfer the soup into a pan over medium heat and cook for about 3–5 minutes or until heated through. Serve immediately with the garnishing of chives and coconut cream.

**Nutrition Info:** Calories 230 Total Fat 8 g Saturated Fat 5.8 g Cholesterol 0 mg Sodium 218 mg Total Carbs 33.5 g Fiber 4.2 g Sugar 27.5 g Protein 8 g

## Balsamic Roasted Carrots

Servings: 4    Cooking Time: 30 Minutes

**Ingredients:**
- 1½ pounds carrots, quartered lengthwise
- 2 tablespoons extra-virgin olive oil
- ¼ teaspoon sea salt
- ⅛ teaspoon freshly ground black pepper
- 3 tablespoons balsamic vinegar

**Directions:**
Preheat the oven to 425°F. In a large bowl, toss the carrots with the olive oil, sea salt, and pepper. Place in a single layer in a roasting pan or on a rimmed baking sheet. Roast for 20 to 30 minutes until the carrots are caramelized. Toss with the vinegar and serve.

**Nutrition Info:** Calories: 132; Protein: 1g; Total Carbohydrates: 17g; Sugars: 8g; Fiber: 4g; Total Fat: 7g; Saturated Fat: 1g; Cholesterol: 0mg; Sodium: 235mg

## Roasted Lemon Mixed Vegetables

Servings: 5    Cooking Time: 20 Minutes

**Ingredients:**
- 2 teaspoons lemon zest
- 1-1/2 cups broccoli florets
- 1-1/2 cups cauliflower florets
- 1 teaspoon oregano, crushed
- ¾ cup red bell pepper, diced
- What you will need from the store cupboard:
- 1 tablespoon olive oil
- 2 sliced garlic cloves
- ¼ teaspoon salt

**Directions:**
Preheat your oven to 350 °F. Bring together the broccoli, garlic, and cauliflower in a baking pan. Drizzle oil. Sprinkle the salt and oregano. Roast for 10 minutes. Now add the bell pepper to the vegetables. Stir and combine. Roast until the vegetables have become light brown and crisp. Sprinkle lemon zest and serve.

**Nutrition Info:** Calories 52, Carbohydrates 5g, Fiber 2g, Cholesterol 0mg, Fat 3g, Sugar 0.2g, Protein 2g, Sodium 134mg

## Butternut Fritters

Servings: 6    Cooking Time: 15 Minutes

**Ingredients:**
- 5 cup butternut squash, grated
- 2 large eggs
- 1 tablespoon. fresh sage, diced fine
- 2/3 cup flour
- 2 tablespoons olive oil
- Salt and pepper, to taste

**Directions:**
Heat oil in a large skillet over med-high heat. In a large bowl, combine squash, eggs, sage and salt and pepper to taste. Fold in flour. Drop ¼ cup mixture into skillet, keeping fritters at least 1 inch apart. Cook till golden brown on both sides, about 2 minutes per side. Transfer to paper towel lined plate. Repeat. Serve immediately with your favorite dipping sauce.

**Nutrition Info:** Calories 164 Total Carbohydrates 24g Net Carbohydrates 21g Protein 4g Fat 6g Sugar 3g Fiber 3g

## Mushroom Toast

Servings: 8    Cooking Time: 10 Minutes

**Ingredients:**
- 1 lb. button mushrooms
- 2 tablespoons thyme, chopped
- 3 tablespoons parsley, chopped
- 2 celery stalks, chopped
- 8 whole-grain bread slices, 1-inch slices
- What you will need from the store cupboard:
- 2 tablespoons sour cream, low-fat
- 1 crushed garlic clove
- ½ cup ricotta cheese
- Pinch of cayenne pepper
- Salt and pepper to taste

**Directions:**
Keep the celery, ricotta, cayenne pepper and parsley in a bowl. Mix well. Preheat your oven to 350 °F. Halve the large mushrooms. Place them in a big skillet. Add

the thyme, garlic, sour cream, and 1 teaspoon of water. Cook covered until your mushrooms have become tender. Season with pepper and salt. In the meantime, toast both sides of the bread slices. Apply ricotta mixture on one side of the toast. Cut it in half. Place toasts on serving plates. Now spoon the mushroom mixture over them before serving.

**Nutrition Info:**Calories 148, Carbohydrates 24g, Fiber 4g, Cholesterol 6mg, Sugar 0.3g, Fat 4g, Protein 8g

## Cauliflower In Vegan Alfredo Sauce

Servings: 1     Cooking Time: 35 Minutes
**Ingredients:**
- Olive oil: 1 tablespoon
- Garlic: 2 cloves
- Vegetable broth: 1 cup
- Sea salt: ½ teaspoon
- Pepper: as per taste
- Chilli flakes: 1 teaspoon
- Onion (diced): 1 medium
- Cauliflower florets (chopped): 4 cups
- Lemon juice (freshly squeezed): 1 teaspoon
- nutritional yeast: 1 tablespoon
- Vegan butter: 2 tablespoons
- Zucchini noodles: for serving

**Directions:**
Begin by positioning a cooking pot on low heat. Stream in the oil and allow it to heat through. Immediately you're done, toss in the chopped onion and set on fire for about 4 minutes. The onion should be translucent. Put in the garlic and Prepare for about 30 seconds. Continuously stir to prevent them from sticking. Put in the vegetable broth and shredded cauliflower florets. Ensure you mix well and cover the stockpot with a lid. Allow the cauliflower cook for 5 minutes and then extract it from the flame. Get a blender and move the cooked cauliflower into it. Palpitate until the puree is smooth and creamy in texture. (Add 1 tablespoon of broth if required for.) Put salt, lemon juice, nutritional yeast, butter, chilli flakes, and pepper to the blender. Mix until all the ingredients fully combine to form a smooth puree. Position the zucchini noodles over a dishing platter and stream the Prepare cauliflower Alfredo sauce over the noodles.

**Nutrition Info:**Fat: 9.1 g Protein: 3.9 g Carbohydrates: 10 g

## Citrus Sautéed Spinach

Servings: 4     Cooking Time: 5 Minutes
**Ingredients:**
- 2 tablespoons extra-virgin olive oil
- 4 cups fresh baby spinach
- 1 teaspoon orange zest
- ¼ cup freshly squeezed orange juice
- ½ teaspoon sea salt
- ⅛ teaspoon freshly ground black pepper

**Directions:**
In a large skillet over medium-high heat, heat the olive oil until it shimmers. Add the spinach and orange zest. Cook for about 3 minutes, stirring occasionally, until the spinach wilts. Stir in the orange juice, sea salt, and pepper. Cook for 2 minutes more, stirring occasionally. Serve hot.

**Nutrition Info:**Calories: 74; Protein: 7g; Total Carbohydrates: 3g; Sugars: 1g; Fiber: 1g; Total Fat: 7g; Saturated Fat: 1g;Cholesterol: 0mg;Sodium: 258mg

## Tempeh With Bell Peppers

Servings: 3     Cooking Time: 15 Minutes
**Ingredients:**
- 2 tablespoons balsamic vinegar
- 2 tablespoons low-sodium soy sauce
- 2 tablespoons tomato sauce
- 1 teaspoon maple syrup
- ½ teaspoon garlic powder
- 1/8 teaspoon red pepper flakes, crushed
- 1 tablespoon vegetable oil
- 8 ounces' tempeh, cut into cubes
- 1 medium onion, chopped
- 2 large green bell peppers, seeded and chopped

**Directions:**
In a small bowl, add the vinegar, soy sauce, tomato sauce, maple syrup, garlic powder, and red pepper flakes and beat until well combined. Set aside. Heat 1 tablespoon of oil in a large skillet over medium heat and cook the tempeh about 2–3 minutes per side. Add the onion and bell peppers and heat for about 2–3 minutes. Stir in the sauce mixture and cook for about 3–5 minutes, stirring frequently. Serve hot.

**Nutrition Info:**Calories 241 Total Fat 13 g Saturated Fat 2.6 g Cholesterol 0 mg Sodium 65 mg Total Carbs 19.7 g Fiber 2.1 g Sugar 8.1 g Protein 16.1 g

## Mushroom Curry

Servings: 3     Cooking Time: 20 Minutes
**Ingredients:**
- 2 cups tomatoes, chopped
- 1 green chili, chopped
- 1 teaspoon fresh ginger, chopped
- ¼ cup cashews
- 2 tablespoons canola oil
- ½ teaspoon cumin seeds
- ¼ teaspoon ground coriander
- ¼ teaspoon ground turmeric
- ¼ teaspoon red chili powder
- 1½ cups fresh shiitake mushrooms, sliced
- 1½ cups fresh button mushrooms, sliced
- 1 cup frozen corn kernels
- 1¼ cups water
- ¼ cup unsweetened coconut milk
- Salt and ground black pepper, to taste

**Directions:**
In a food processor, add the tomatoes, green chili, ginger, and cashews, and pulse until a smooth paste forms. In a pan, heat the oil over medium heat and sauté the cumin seeds for about 1 minute. Add the spices and sauté for about 1 minute. Add the tomato paste and cook for about 5 minutes. Stir in the mushrooms, corn, water, and coconut milk, and bring to a boil. Cook for about 10–12 minutes, stirring occasionally. Season with salt and black pepper and remove from the heat. Serve hot.

**Nutrition Info:**Calories 311 Total Fat 20.4 g Saturated Fat 6.1 g Cholesterol 0 mg Sodium 244 mg Total Carbs 32g Fiber 5.6 g Sugar 9 g Protein 8 g

## Bean Medley Chili

Servings: 8     Cooking Time: 20 Minutes
**Ingredients:**
- 1 can black beans, rinsed and drained
- 1 can garbanzo beans, rinsed and drained
- 1 teaspoon cumin, ground
- ¼ cup cilantro, snipped
- 2 onions, chopped
- What you will need from the store cupboard:
- 1 can chicken broth
- 3 tablespoons of chili powder
- 1 can chipotle chili pepper in adobo sauce
- ¼ teaspoon salt

**Directions:**
Bring together the beans, pepper, onion, chili powder, salt, and cumin in your cooker.     Add the broth. Cover and cook.     Stir the cilantro in.     You can serve it with rice if desired.
**Nutrition Info:**Calories 191, Carbohydrates 38g, Cholesterol 0mg, Fiber 12g, Fat 2g, Protein 12g, Sugar 0.7g, Sodium 659mg

## Roasted Carrots

Servings: 4     Cooking Time: 20 Minutes
**Ingredients:**
- 2 tablespoons olive oil, divided
- 2 tablespoons balsamic vinegar
- 1 tablespoon pure maple syrup
- 1 lb. carrots, sliced into small pieces
- Salt to taste
- 2 tablespoons hazelnuts, chopped

**Directions:**
Preheat your oven to 400 degrees F.     Combine 1 tablespoon oil with vinegar and maple syrup.     Set aside the mixture.     In another bowl, toss the carrots in remaining oil and season with salt.     Arrange on a single layer in a baking pan.     Roast for 15 minutes. Pour the reserved mixture over the carrots and mix. Roast for additional 5 minutes.     Sprinkle hazelnuts on top before serving.
**Nutrition Info:**Calories 130 Total Fat 7 g Saturated Fat 1g Cholesterol 0 mg Sodium 226 mg Total Carbohydrate 16 g Dietary Fiber 3 g Total Sugars 10 g Protein 1 g Potassium 382 mg

## Boiled Potatoes With Tomato Salsa

Servings: 8     Cooking Time: 15 Minutes
**Ingredients:**
- 6 potatoes, sliced into wedges
- 1 clove garlic, minced
- 3 large tomatoes, diced
- 2 tablespoons white onion, chopped
- 2 teaspoons fresh marjoram, chopped
- Salt and pepper to taste

**Directions:**

Boil the potatoes until soft enough to poke with a fork. Combine the rest of the ingredients in a bowl.     Serve potatoes with salsa.
**Nutrition Info:**Calories 200 Total Fat 10 g Saturated Fat 1 g Cholesterol 25 mg Sodium 81 mg Total Carbohydrate 10 g Dietary Fiber 5 g Total Sugars 1 g Protein 25 g Potassium 560 mg

## Lentil And Eggplant Stew

Servings: 2     Cooking Time: 35 Minutes
**Ingredients:**
- 1lb eggplant
- 1lb dry lentils
- 1 cup chopped vegetables
- 1 cup low sodium vegetable broth

**Directions:**
Mix all the ingredients in your Instant Pot.     Cook on Stew for 35 minutes.     Release the pressure naturally.
**Nutrition Info:**Calories: 310 Carbs: 22 Sugar: 6 Fat: 10 Protein: 32 GL: 16

## Asian Fried Eggplant

Servings: 4     Cooking Time: 40 Minutes
**Ingredients:**
- 1 large eggplant, sliced into fourths
- 3 green onions, diced, green tips only
- 1 teaspoon fresh ginger, peeled & diced fine
- ¼ cup + 1 teaspoon cornstarch
- 1 ½ tablespoon. soy sauce
- 1 ½ tablespoon. sesame oil
- 1 tablespoon. vegetable oil
- 1 tablespoon. fish sauce
- 2 teaspoon Splenda
- ¼ teaspoon salt

**Directions:**
Place eggplant on paper towels and sprinkle both sides with salt. Let for 1 hour to remove excess moisture. Pat dry with more paper towels.     In a small bowl, whisk together soy sauce, sesame oil, fish sauce, Splenda, and 1 teaspoon cornstarch.     Coat both sides of the eggplant with the ¼ cup cornstarch, use more if needed.     Heat oil in a large skillet, over med-high heat. Add ½ the ginger and 1 green onion, then lay 2 slices of eggplant on top. Use ½ the sauce mixture to lightly coat both sides of the eggplant. Cook 8-10 minutes per side. Repeat. Serve garnished with remaining green onions.
**Nutrition Info:**Calories 155 Total Carbohydrates 18g Net Carbohydrates 13g Protein 2g Fat 9g Sugar 6g Fiber 5g

## Carrot Cake Bites

Servings: 22     Cooking Time: 15 Minutes
**Ingredients:**
- 4 oz. carrots, chopped
- ¼ cup chia seeds
- ¼ cup pecans, chopped
- ¼ teaspoon turmeric, ground
- ¾ teaspoon cinnamon, ground
- What you will need from the store cupboard:
- 1 teaspoon vanilla extract

- 1 cup pitted dates
- ¼ teaspoon salt
- Pinch of ground pepper

**Directions:**
Bring together the chia seeds, pecans, and dates in your food processor. Pulse until everything is chopped and well combined. Now add the vanilla, carrots, cinnamon, salt, pepper, and turmeric. Process until you see a paste starting to form. Create small balls by rolling this mixture.

**Nutrition Info:**Calories 48, Carbohydrates 8g, Fiber 2g, Cholesterol 0mg, Fat 2g, Sugar 0.5g, Protein 1g, Sodium 30mg

## Broccoli With Ginger And Garlic

Servings: 4     Cooking Time: 11 Minutes
**Ingredients:**
- 2 tablespoons extra-virgin olive oil
- 2 cups broccoli florets
- 1 tablespoon grated fresh ginger
- ½ teaspoon sea salt
- ⅛ teaspoon freshly ground black pepper
- 3 garlic cloves, minced

**Directions:**
In a large skillet over medium-high heat, heat the olive oil until it shimmers. Add the broccoli, ginger, sea salt, and pepper. Cook for about 10 minutes, stirring occasionally, until the broccoli is soft and starts to brown. Add the garlic and cook for 30 seconds, stirring constantly. Remove from the heat and serve.

**Nutrition Info:**Per Serving Calories: 80; Protein: 1g; Total Carbohydrates: 4g; Sugars: 1g; Fiber: 1g; Total Fat: 0g; Saturated Fat: 1g; Cholesterol: 0mg; Sodium: 249mg

## Barley Pilaf

Servings: 4     Cooking Time: 1 Hour 5 Minutes
**Ingredients:**
- ½ cup pearl barley
- 1 cup low-sodium vegetable broth
- 2 tablespoons olive oil, divided
- 2 garlic cloves, minced finely
- ½ cup onion, chopped
- ½ cup eggplant, sliced thinly
- ½ cup green bell pepper, seeded and chopped
- ½ cup red bell pepper, seeded and chopped
- 2 tablespoons fresh cilantro, chopped
- 2 tablespoons fresh mint leaves, chopped

**Directions:**
In a pan, add the barley and broth over medium-high heat and bring to a boil. Immediately, reduce the heat to low and simmer, covered for about 45 minutes or until all the liquid is absorbed. In a large skillet, heat 1 tablespoon of oil over high heat and sauté the garlic for about 1 minute. Stir in the cooked barley and cook for about 3 minutes. Remove from heat and set aside. In another skillet, heat remaining oil over medium heat and sauté the onion for about 5-7 minutes. Add the eggplant and bell peppers and stir fry for about 3 minutes. Stir in the remaining ingredients except walnuts and cook for about 2-3 minutes. Stir in barley mixture and

cook for about 2-3 minutes. Serve hot. Meal Prep Tip: Transfer the pilaf into a large bowl and set aside to cool. Divide the pilaf into 4 containers evenly. Cover the containers and refrigerate for 1 day. Reheat in the microwave before serving.

**Nutrition Info:**Calories 168 Total Fat 7.4 g Saturated Fat 1.1 g Cholesterol 0 mg Total Carbs 23.5 g Sugar 1.9 g Fiber 5 g Sodium 22 mg Potassium 164 mg Protein 3.6 g

## Kale With Miso & Ginger

Servings: 6     Cooking Time: 10 Minutes
**Ingredients:**
- 8 oz. fresh kale, sliced into strips
- 1 clove garlic, minced
- 1 tablespoon lime juice
- ½ teaspoon lime zest
- 2 tablespoons oil
- 2 tablespoons rice vinegar
- 1 teaspoon fresh ginger, grated
- 2 teaspoons miso
- 2 tablespoons dry roasted cashews, chopped

**Directions:**
Steam kale on a steamer basket in a pot with water. Transfer kale to a bowl. Mix the rest of the ingredients except cashews in another bowl. Toss kale in the mixture. Top with chopped cashews before serving.

**Nutrition Info:**Calories 86 Total Fat 5 g Saturated Fat 0 g Cholesterol 0 mg Sodium 104 mg Total Carbohydrate 9 g Dietary Fiber 2 g Total Sugars 2 g Protein 3 g Potassium 352 mg

## Beans, Walnuts & Veggie Burgers

Servings: 8     Cooking Time: 25 Minutes
**Ingredients:**
- ½ cup walnuts
- 1 carrot, peeled and chopped
- 1 celery stalk, chopped
- 4 scallions, chopped
- 5 garlic cloves, chopped
- 2¼ cups cooked black beans
- 2½ cups sweet potato, peeled and grated
- ½ teaspoon red pepper flakes, crushed
- ¼ teaspoon cayenne pepper
- Salt and ground black pepper, as required

**Directions:**
Preheat the oven to 400 degrees F. Line a baking sheet with parchment paper. In a food processor, add walnuts and pulse until finely ground. Add the carrot, celery, scallion and garlic and pulse until chopped finely. Transfer the vegetable mixture into a large bowl. In the same food processor, add beans and pulse until chopped. Add 1½ cups of sweet potato and pulse until a chunky mixture forms. Transfer the bean mixture into the bowl with vegetable mixture. Stir in the remaining sweet potato and spices and mix until well combined. Make 8 patties from mixture. Arrange the patties onto prepared baking sheet in a single layer. Bake for about 25 minutes. Serve hot. Meal Prep Tip: Remove the burgers from oven and set aside to cool completely. Store these burgers in an airtight container, by placing parchment papers between the burgers to

avoid the sticking. These burgers can be stored in the freezer for up to 3 weeks. Before serving, thaw the burgers and then reheat in microwave.
**Nutrition Info:**Calories 177 Total Fat 5 g Saturated Fat 0.3 g Cholesterol 0 mg Total Carbs 27.6 g Sugar 5.3 g Fiber 7.6 g Sodium 205 mg Potassium 398 mg Protein 8 g

## Artichoke Quiche

Servings: 6     Cooking Time: 15 Minutes
**Ingredients:**
- 2 cups long-grain rice, cooked
- ¾ cup egg substitute
- ¼ cup green onions, sliced
- ¼ teaspoon white pepper, ground
- 1 can artichoke hearts
- What you will need from the store cupboard:
- ¾ cup low-fat cheddar cheese
- 1 garlic clove, crushed
- ¾ cup fat-free milk
- ½ teaspoon salt
- 1 tablespoon Dijon mustard
- Cooking spray

**Directions:**
Bring together the egg substitute, ¼ cup cheese, garlic, salt, and rice.     Apply cooking spray to a pie plate. Bake for 5 minutes.     Keep the artichoke quarters at the bottom of your rice crust.     Now sprinkle the remaining cheese.     Combine the remaining milk, egg substitute, and the other ingredients.     Pour the cheese over. Bake until it sets.     Cut into wedges and garnish with the onion strips.
**Nutrition Info:**Calories 169, Carbohydrates 23g, Fiber 1g, Cholesterol 11mg, Fat 4g, Protein 10g, Sodium 490mg

## Quinoa In Tomato Sauce

Servings: 4     Cooking Time: 40 Minutes
**Ingredients:**
- 2 tablespoons olive oil
- 1 cup quinoa, rinsed
- 1 green bell pepper, seeded and chopped
- 1 medium onion, chopped finely
- 3 garlic cloves, minced
- 2½ cups filtered water
- 2 cups tomatoes, crushed finely
- 1 teaspoon red chili powder
- ¼ teaspoon ground cumin
- ¼ teaspoon garlic powder
- Ground black pepper, as required

**Directions:**
In a large pan, heat the oil over medium-high heat and cook the quinoa, onion, bell pepper and garlic for about 5 minutes, stirring frequently.     Stir in the remaining ingredients and bring to a boil.     Now, reduce the heat to medium-low.     Cover the pan tightly and simmer for about 30 minutes, stirring occasionally.     Serve hot. Meal Prep Tip: Transfer the quinoa mixture into a large bowl and set aside to cool. Divide the chili into 4 containers evenly. Cover the containers and refrigerate for 1-2 days. Reheat in the microwave before serving.

**Nutrition Info:**Calories 260 Total Fat 10 g Saturated Fat 1.4 g Cholesterol 0 mg Total Carbs 36.9 g Sugar 5.2 g Fiber 5.4 g Sodium 16 mg Potassium 575 mg Protein 7.7 g

## Black Bean With Poblano Tortilla Wraps

Servings: 4     Cooking Time: 10 Minutes
**Ingredients:**
- ½ teaspoon cumin, ground
- 1/3 cup poblano chili, chopped
- 1 cup avocado, diced and peeled
- ¼ cup red onion, chopped
- 1 can rinse and drained black beans
- What you will need from the store cupboard:
- ½ cup low-fat sour cream
- 3 tablespoons lime juice
- 4 flour tortillas
- ¼ teaspoon salt

**Directions:**
Combine the cumin and sour cream in a bowl. Use a whisk to stir.     Bring together the beans and other ingredients.     Spoon out the mixture at the center of the tortillas.     Roll them up. Cut through the middle. Use wooden picks to secure.     Serve with your sour cream mixture.
**Nutrition Info:**Calories 298, Carbohydrates 40g, Fiber 5g, Cholesterol 16mg, Fat 13g, Protein 9g, Sodium 606mg

## Mixed Greens Salad

Servings: 6     Cooking Time: 0 Minutes
**Ingredients:**
- 6 cups mixed salad greens
- 1 cup cucumber, chopped
- ½ cup carrot, shredded
- ¼ cup bell pepper, sliced into strips
- ¼ cup cherry tomatoes, sliced in half
- 6 tablespoons white onion, chopped
- 6 tablespoons balsamic vinaigrette dressing

**Directions:**
Toss all the ingredients in a large salad bowl.     Drizzle dressing on top or serve on the side.
**Nutrition Info:**Calories 23 Total Fat 1 g Saturated Fat 0 g Cholesterol 0 mg Sodium 138 mg Total Carbohydrate 4 g Dietary Fiber 1 g Total Sugars 1 g Protein 1 g Potassium 142 mg

## Tofu Curry

Servings: 2     Cooking Time: 20 Minutes
**Ingredients:**
- 2 cups cubed extra firm tofu
- 2 cups mixed stir fry vegetables
- 0.5 cup soy yogurt
- 3tbsp curry paste
- 1tbsp oil or ghee

**Directions:**
Set the Instant Pot to saute and add the oil and curry paste.     When the onion is soft, add the remaining ingredients except the yogurt and seal.     Cook on Stew

for 20 minutes.    Release the pressure naturally and serve with a scoop of soy yogurt.
**Nutrition Info:**Calories: 300 Carbs: 9 Sugar: 4 Fat: 14 Protein: 42 GL: 7

## Baked Beans

Servings: 6    Cooking Time: 20 Minutes
**Ingredients:**
- 2 cups navy beans, overnight soaked in cold water
- 2/3 cups green bell pepper, diced
- 1 can tomatoes, diced
- 1 onion, sliced
- What you will need from the store cupboard:
- 3 tablespoons molasses
- ¼ cup of orange juice
- ¼ cup maple syrup
- 1 tablespoon Worcestershire sauce
- 1/4 teaspoon mustard powder
- 2 tablespoons stevia sugar
- 2 tablespoons salt

**Directions:**
Preheat your oven to 350 °F    Simmer the beans. Drain and keep the liquid.    Place beans in a casserole dish with the onion.    Bring together the dry mustard, pepper, salt, molasses, Worcestershire sauce, tomatoes, sugar substitute and orange juice in your saucepan. Boil the mix. Pour over your beans.    Pour the reserved bean water, covering the beans.    Use aluminum foil to cover the dish.    Now bake in the oven. The beans must get tender.    Remove the foil and add some liquid if needed.
**Nutrition Info:**Calories 482, Carbohydrates 65g, Cholesterol 25mg, Fiber 12g, Fat 16g, Protein 21g, Sugar 2.2g, Sodium 512mg

## Spicy Black Beans

Servings: 6    Cooking Time: 1½ Hours
**Ingredients:**
- 4 cups filtered water
- 1½ cups dried black beans, soaked for 8 hours and drained
- ½ teaspoon ground turmeric
- 3 tablespoons olive oil
- 1 small onion, chopped finely
- 1 green chili, chopped
- 1 (1-inch) piece fresh ginger, minced
- 2 garlic cloves, minced
- 1-1½ tablespoons ground coriander
- 1 teaspoon ground cumin
- ½ teaspoon cayenne pepper
- Sea salt, as required
- 2 medium tomatoes, chopped finely
- ½ cup fresh cilantro, chopped

**Directions:**
In a large pan, add water, black beans and turmeric and bring to a boil on high heat.    Now, reduce the heat to low and simmer, covered for about 1 hour or till desired doneness of beans.    Meanwhile, in a skillet, heat the oil over medium heat and sauté the onion for about 4-5 minutes.    Add the green chili, ginger, garlic, spices and salt and sauté for about 1-2 minutes.    Stir in the

tomatoes and cook for about 10 minutes, stirring occasionally.    Transfer the tomato mixture into the pan with black beans and stir to combine.    Increase the heat to medium-low and simmer for about 15-20 minutes.    Stir in the cilantro and simmer for about 5 minutes.    Serve hot.    Meal Prep Tip: Transfer the beans mixture into a large bowl and set aside to cool. Divide the mixture into 6 containers evenly. Cover the containers and refrigerate for 1-2 days. Reheat in the microwave before serving.
**Nutrition Info:**Calories 160 Total Fat 8 g Saturated Fat 1 g Cholesterol 0 mg Total Carbs 17.9 g Sugar 2.4 g Fiber 6.2 g Sodium 50 mg Potassium 343 mg Protein 6 g

## Cauliflower Mushroom Risotto

Servings: 2    Cooking Time: 30 Minutes
**Ingredients:**
- 1 medium head cauliflower, grated
- 8-ounce Porcini mushrooms, sliced
- 1 yellow onion, diced fine
- 2 cup low sodium vegetable broth
- 2 teaspoon garlic, diced fine
- 2 teaspoon white wine vinegar
- Salt & pepper, to taste
- Olive oil cooking spray

**Directions:**
Heat oven to 350 degrees. Line a baking sheet with foil. Place the mushrooms on the prepared pan and spray with cooking spray. Sprinkle with salt and toss to coat. Bake 10-12 minutes, or until golden brown and the mushrooms start to crisp.    Spray a large skillet with cooking spray and place over med-high heat. Add onion and cook, stirring frequently, until translucent, about 3-4 minutes. Add garlic and cook 2 minutes, until golden. Add the cauliflower and cook 1 minute, stirring.    Place the broth in a saucepan and bring to a simmer. Add to the skillet, ¼ cup at a time, mixing well after each addition.    Stir in vinegar. Reduce heat to low and let simmer, 4-5 minutes, or until most of the liquid has evaporated.    Spoon cauliflower mixture onto plates, or in bowls, and top with mushrooms. Serve.
**Nutrition Info:**Calories 134 Total Carbohydrates 22g Protein 10g Fat 0g Sugar 5g Fiber 2g

## Tofu With Peas

Servings: 5    Cooking Time: 20 Minutes
**Ingredients:**
- 1 tablespoon chili-garlic sauce
- 3 tablespoons low-sodium soy sauce
- 2 tablespoons canola oil, divided
- 1 (16-ounce) package extra-firm tofu, drained, pressed, and cubed
- 1 cup yellow onion, chopped
- 1 tablespoon fresh ginger, minced
- 2 garlic cloves, minced
- 2 large tomatoes, chopped finely
- 5 cups frozen peas, thawed
- 1 teaspoon white sesame seeds

**Directions:**

For sauce: in a bowl, add the chili-garlic sauce and soy sauce and mix until well combined.    In a large skillet, heat 1 tablespoon of oil over medium-high heat and cook the tofu for about 4–5 minutes or until browned completely, stirring occasionally.    Transfer the tofu into a bowl.    In the same skillet, heat the remaining oil over medium heat and sauté the onion for about 3–4 minutes.    Add the ginger and garlic and sauté for about 1 minute.    Add the tomatoes and cook for about 4–5 minutes, crushing with the back of spoon.    Stir in all three peas and cook for about 2–3 minutes.    Stir in the sauce mixture and tofu and cook for about 1–2 minutes.    Serve hot with the garnishing of sesame seeds.

**Nutrition Info:**Calories 291 Total Fat 11.9 g Saturated Fat 1.1 g Cholesterol 0 mg Sodium 732 mg Total Carbs 31.6 g Fiber 10.8 g Sugar 11.5 g Protein 19 g

## Cauliflower And Kabocha Squash Soup

Servings: 1     Cooking Time: 35 Minutes
**Ingredients:**
- Olive oil: 2 tablespoons
- Garlic (minced): 3 cloves
- Cauliflower florets: 2½ cups
- Ground cardamom: ½ teaspoon
- Bay leaves: 2
- Vanilla almond milk (unsweetened): ½ cup
- Pepper: ¼ teaspoon
- Yellow onion (diced): ½
- Fresh ginger (minced): 1 tablespoon
- Kabocha squash (cubed): 2½ cups
- Cayenne: ¼ teaspoon
- Vegetable broth: 4 cups
- Salt: ½ teaspoon

**Directions:**
Begin by streaming the olive oil into a nonstick saucepan and position it over a high flame.    Toss in the onion, ginger, and garlic. Sauté for around 3 minutes.    Then put in the squash, cauliflower, cayenne, bay leaves, and cardamom. Combine well.    Stream in the vegetable broth and take the vegetables and stock mixture to a boil. Reduce the flame and allow the soup simmer for 10 minutes.    Extract the pan and use the blender to puree the mixture.    Immediately the soup is pureed, replace the pan to the low heat. Put in the almond milk. Combine well.    Finalize by spicing with pepper and salt.

**Nutrition Info:**Fat: 7.7 g Protein: 3.4 g Carbohydrates: 11.6 g

## Mango Tofu Curry

Servings: 2     Cooking Time: 35 Minutes
**Ingredients:**
- 1lb cubed extra firm tofu
- 1lb chopped vegetables
- 1 cup low carb mango sauce
- 1 cup vegetable broth
- 2tbsp curry paste

**Directions:**
Mix all the ingredients in your Instant Pot.    Cook on Stew for 35 minutes.    Release the pressure naturally.

**Nutrition Info:**Calories: 310 Carbs: 20 Sugar: 9 Fat: 4 Protein: 37 GL: 19

## Banana Curry

Servings: 3     Cooking Time: 15 Minutes
**Ingredients:**
- 2 tablespoons olive
- 2 yellow onions, chopped
- 8 garlic cloves, minced
- 2 tablespoons curry powder
- 1 tablespoon ground ginger
- 1 tablespoon ground cumin
- 1 teaspoon ground turmeric
- 1 teaspoon ground cinnamon
- 1 teaspoon red chili powder
- Salt and ground black pepper, to taste
- 2/3 cup soy yogurt
- 1 cup tomato puree
- 2 bananas, peeled and sliced
- 3 tomatoes, chopped finely
- ¼ cup unsweetened coconut flakes

**Directions:**
In a large pan, heat the oil over medium heat and sauté onion for about 4–5 minutes.    Add the garlic, curry powder, and spices, and sauté for about 1 minute.    Add the soy yogurt and tomato sauce and bring to a gentle boil.    Stir in the bananas and simmer for about 3 minutes.    Stir in the tomatoes and simmer for about 1–2 minutes.    Stir in the coconut flakes and immediately remove from the heat.    Serve hot.

**Nutrition Info:**Calories 382 Total Fat 18.2 g Saturated Fat 6.6 g Cholesterol 0 mg Sodium 108 mg Total Carbs 53.4 g Fiber 11.3 g Sugar 24.8 g Protein 9 g

## Dried Fruit Squash

Servings: 4     Cooking Time: 40 Minutes
**Ingredients:**
- ¼ cup water
- 1 medium butternut squash, halved and seeded
- ½ tablespoon olive oil
- ½ tablespoon balsamic vinegar
- Salt and ground black pepper, to taste
- 4 large dates, pitted and chopped
- 4 fresh figs, chopped
- 3 tablespoons pistachios, chopped
- 2 tablespoons pumpkin seeds

**Directions:**
Preheat the oven to 375°F.    Place the water in the bottom of a baking dish.    Arrange the squash halves in a large baking dish, hollow-side up, and drizzle with oil and vinegar.    Sprinkle with salt and black pepper. Spread the dates, figs, and pistachios on top.    Bake for about 40 minutes, or until squash becomes tender. Serve hot with the garnishing of pumpkin seeds.

**Nutrition Info:**Calories 227 Total Fat 5.5 g Saturated Fat 0.8 g Cholesterol 0 mg Sodium 66 mg Total Carbs 46.4 g Fiber 7.5 g Sugar 19.6 g Protein 5 g

## Fake On-stew

Servings: 2     Cooking Time: 25 Minutes

**Ingredients:**
- 0.5lb soy bacon
- 1lb chopped vegetables
- 1 cup low sodium vegetable broth
- 1tbsp nutritional yeast

**Directions:**
Mix all the ingredients in your Instant Pot. Cook on Stew for 25 minutes. Release the pressure naturally.

**Nutrition Info:**Calories: 200 Carbs: 12 Sugar: 3 Fat: 7 Protein: 41 GL: 5

## Squash Medley

Servings: 2    Cooking Time: 20 Minutes.

**Ingredients:**
- 2lbs mixed squash
- 0.5 cup mixed veg
- 1 cup vegetable stock
- 2tbsp olive oil
- 2tbsp mixed herbs

**Directions:**
Put the squash in the steamer basket and add the stock into the Instant Pot. Steam the squash in your Instant Pot for 10 minutes. Depressurize and pour away the remaining stock. Set to saute and add the oil and remaining ingredients. Cook until a light crust forms.

**Nutrition Info:**Calories: 100 Carbs: 10 Sugar: 3 Fat: 6 Protein: 5 GL: 20

## Porcini Mushrooms & Eggplant

Servings: 6    Cooking Time: 30 Minutes

**Ingredients:**
- 1 lb. eggplant, cubed
- 2 tablespoons olive oil
- Salt and pepper to taste
- ½ oz. dried porcini mushrooms
- 1 cup boiling water
- ⅓ cup balsamic vinegar
- 1 teaspoon fresh thyme, chopped
- ½ cup cherry tomatoes, sliced in half
- 1 tablespoon fresh basil, chopped

**Directions:**
Preheat your oven to 425 degrees F. Arrange the eggplant cubes on a baking pan. Drizzle oil on top and season with salt and pepper. Roast for 15 minutes. While waiting, soak mushrooms in hot water. Let it sit for 15 minutes. Drain water, and then chop. Pour the vinegar in a saucepan over medium heat. Bring to a boil and then reduce heat to simmer for 5 minutes. Add the mushrooms and fresh thyme. Drizzle balsamic mixture on top of the eggplants and serve with the tomatoes with basil.

**Nutrition Info:**Calories 77 Total Fat 5 g Saturated Fat 1 g Cholesterol 0 mg Sodium 103 mg Total Carbohydrate 8 g Dietary Fiber 3 g Total Sugars 4 g Protein 1 g Potassium 232 mg

## Roasted Asparagus With Lemon And Pine Nuts

Servings: 4    Cooking Time: 20 Minutes

**Ingredients:**

- 1-pound asparagus, trimmed
- 2 tablespoons extra-virgin olive oil
- Juice of 1 lemon
- Zest of 1 lemon
- ¼ cup pine nuts
- ½ teaspoon sea salt
- ⅛ teaspoon freshly ground black pepper

**Directions:**
Preheat the oven to 425°F. In a large bowl, toss the asparagus with the olive oil, lemon juice and zest, pine nuts, sea salt, and pepper. Spread in a roasting pan in an even layer. Roast for about 20 minutes until the asparagus is browned.

**Nutrition Info:**Calories: 144; Protein: 4g; Total Carbohydrates: 6g; Sugars: 3g; Fiber: 3g; Total Fat: 13g;Saturated Fat: 1g; Cholesterol: 0mg; Sodium: 240mg

## Veggie Stew

Servings: 3    Cooking Time: 30 Minutes

**Ingredients:**
- 2 tablespoons olive oil
- 1 large onion, chopped
- 2 garlic cloves, minced
- ¼ teaspoon fresh ginger, grated finely
- 1 teaspoon ground cumin
- 1 teaspoon cayenne pepper
- Salt and ground black pepper, to taste
- 2 cups homemade vegetable broth
- 1½ cups small broccoli florets
- 1½ cups small cauliflower florets
- 1 tablespoon fresh lemon juice
- 1 cup cashews
- 1 teaspoon fresh lemon zest, grated finely

**Directions:**
In a large soup pan, heat oil over medium heat and sauté the onion for about 3–4 minutes. Add the garlic, ginger, and spices and sauté for about 1 minute. Add 1 cup of the broth and bring to a boil. Add the vegetables and again bring to a boil. Cover the soup pan and cook for about 15–20 minutes, stirring occasionally. Stir in the lemon juice and remove from the heat. Serve hot with the topping of cashews and lemon zest.

**Nutrition Info:**Calories 425 Total Fat 32 g Saturated Fat 5.9 g Cholesterol 0 mg Sodium 601 mg Total Carbs 27.6 g Fiber 5.2 g Sugar 7.1 g Protein 13.4 g

## Spiced Couscous Tomatoes

Servings: 8    Cooking Time: 15 Minutes

**Ingredients:**
- ½ teaspoon cumin, ground
- 1 teaspoon coriander, ground
- 8 beefsteak tomatoes
- ½ cup sliced almonds
- 1 eggplant, cut into ½ inch slices
- What you will need from the store cupboard:
- 1 cup vegetable broth, low-sodium
- 1 tablespoon olive oil
- ½ cup couscous
- 1 teaspoon harissa paste

- Salt and pepper to taste
- Pinch of ground cinnamon

**Directions:**
Sprinkle some salt inside the hollowed-out tomatoes. Keep them on a plate, upside down. Use paper towels to cover. Heat ½ of the olive oil in your saucepan. Add almonds. Cook for 2-3 minutes over low temperature. Add the other ingredients to the saucepan. Stir the eggplant in. Cook while turning until it is tender and brown. Stir in the cumin, cinnamon, and coriander. Pour the broth in and boil. Now add the couscous. Take out from the heat. Keep aside for 5 minutes. Return to low temperature. Cook for 2 minutes. Use a fork, separating the couscous grains. Stir the almonds in and add the harissa paste to the mix. Pour over the couscous. Season with pepper. Mix well. Spoon the mixture into your tomatoes.

**Nutrition Info:** Calories 175, Fat 6g, Protein 5g, Carbohydrates 28g, Fiber 5g, Cholesterol 0mg, Sugar 1.1g

## Black Bean And Veggie Soup Topped With Lime Salsa

Servings: 1    Cooking Time: 35 Minutes

**Ingredients:**
- Onions (diced): 2
- Celery (diced): 3 sticks
- Garlic (finely chopped): 3 cloves
- Cilantro: ½ bunch
- Dried oregano: 1 tablespoon
- Sea salt: ½ tablespoon
- Boiling water: 1 quart
- Salad onion (finely chopped): ½ small
- Carrots (diced): 2
- Red bell peppers (diced): 2
- Red chilis (remove seed): 2
- Bay leaf: 1
- Black pepper (freshly ground): 1 tablespoon
- Black beans (drained and rinsed): 2 cans (15 ounces)
- Tomato (finely chopped): 1
- Fresh juice of ½ lime

**Directions:**
Begin by extracting the leaves and stalks from the cilantro. Neatly shred the stalks and leaves. Arrange aside Ge a large saucepan and stream in 3 tablespoons of water. In this, put the carrots, onions, bell peppers, celery, red chillies, garlic, coriander stalks, oregano, bay leaf, sea salt, and pepper. Mix until well-combined. Cover the pan using a lid and allow the veggies to cook for about 10 minutes. Keep mixing. Put the black beans and boiling water into the saucepan. Keep stirring. Extract the lid from the saucepan and low heat. Allow the soup to cook for half a minute. While the soup is on a high flame, form the lime salsa. In this, you will mix the tomato, salad onion, and cilantro leaves in a small bowl. Crush in the fresh lime juice. Stream the soup in a big and deep bowl and finish by topping with lime salsa.

**Nutrition Info:** Fat: 2.4 g Protein: 17.2 g Carbohydrates: 53.9 g

## Chili Sin Carne

Servings: 2    Cooking Time: 35 Minutes

**Ingredients:**
- 3 cups mixed cooked beans
- 2 cups chopped tomatoes
- 1tbsp yeast extract
- 2 squares very dark chocolate
- 1tbsp red chili flakes

**Directions:**
Mix all the ingredients in your Instant Pot. Cook on Beans for 35 minutes. Release the pressure naturally.

**Nutrition Info:** Calories: 240 Carbs: 20 Sugar: 5 Fat: 3 Protein: 36 GL: 11

## 3-veggie Combo

Servings: 4    Cooking Time: 25 Minutes

**Ingredients:**
- 1 tablespoon olive oil
- 1 small yellow onion, chopped
- 1 teaspoon fresh thyme, chopped
- 1 garlic clove, minced
- 8 ounces' fresh button mushroom, sliced
- 1 pound Brussels sprouts
- 3 cups fresh spinach
- 4 tablespoons walnuts
- Salt and ground black pepper, to taste

**Directions:**
In a large skillet, heat the oil over medium heat and sauté the onion for about 3–4 minutes. Add the thyme and garlic and sauté for about 1 minute. Add the mushrooms and cook for about 15 minutes, or until caramelized. Add the Brussels sprouts and cook for about 2–3 minutes. Stir in the spinach and cook for about 3–4 minutes. Stir in the walnuts, salt, and black pepper, and remove from the heat. Serve hot.

**Nutrition Info:** Calories 153 Total Fat 8.8 g Saturated Fat 0.9 g Cholesterol 0 mg Sodium 94 mg Total Carbs 15.8 g Fiber 6.3 g Sugar 4.4 g Protein 8.5 g

## Lentil And Chickpea Curry

Servings: 2    Cooking Time: 20 Minutes

**Ingredients:**
- 2 cups dry lentils and chickpeas
- 1 thinly sliced onion
- 1 cup chopped tomato
- 3tbsp curry paste
- 1tbsp oil or ghee

**Directions:**
Set the Instant Pot to saute and add the onion, oil, and curry paste. When the onion is soft, add the remaining ingredients and seal. Cook on Stew for 20 minutes. Release the pressure naturally.

**Nutrition Info:** Calories: 360 Carbs: 26 Sugar: 6 Fat: 19 Protein: 23 GL: 10

## Pea And Mint Soup

Servings: 2    Cooking Time: 35 Minutes

**Ingredients:**
- 1lb green peas
- 2 cups low sodium vegetable broth

- 3tbsp mint sauce

**Directions:**
Mix all the ingredients in your Instant Pot.    Cook on Stew for 35 minutes.    Release the pressure naturally. Blend into a rough soup.

**Nutrition Info:** Calories: 130 Carbs: 17 Sugar: 4 Fat: 5 Protein: 19 GL: 11

## Kale & Tofu Salad

Servings: 4    Cooking Time: 15 Minutes

**Ingredients:**
- 1 block tofu, sliced into cubes
- ¼ cup Worcestershire sauce
- ¼ cup freshly squeezed lemon juice
- 1 teaspoon onion powder
- 1 teaspoon garlic powder
- 3 teaspoons olive oil
- 8 cups kale, chopped
- ¼ cup nutritional yeast
- ¼ cup pumpkin seeds, toasted
- ½ cup Caesar dressing
- 1 avocado, sliced

**Directions:**
Dry the tofu with paper towel.    In a bowl, mix the Worcestershire sauce, lemon juice, onion powder and garlic powder.    Coat the tofu with this mixture.    Let it stand for 15 minutes.    Discard the marinade. Pour the oil in a pan over medium heat.    Cook the tofu until golden brown on all sides.    Drain the oil and set aside.    In a bowl, toss the kale in nutritional yeast. Divide into containers.    Top each container with croutons and pumpkin seeds.    Pour dressing on top and serve with avocado slices.

**Nutrition Info:** Calories 400 Total Fat 28 g Saturated Fat 4 g Cholesterol 6 mg Sodium 423 mg Total Carbohydrate 19 g Dietary Fiber 9 g Total Sugars 2 g Protein 20 g Potassium 670 mg

## Tofu With Brussels Sprouts

Servings: 3    Cooking Time: 15 Minutes

**Ingredients:**
- 1½ tablespoons olive oil, divided
- 8 ounces' extra-firm tofu, drained, pressed, and cut into slices
- 2 garlic cloves, chopped
- 1/3 cup pecans, toasted, and chopped
- 1 tablespoon unsweetened applesauce
- ¼ cup fresh cilantro, chopped
- ½ pound Brussels sprouts, trimmed and cut into wide ribbons
- ¾ pound mixed bell peppers, seeded and sliced

**Directions:**
In a skillet, heat ½ tablespoon of the oil over medium heat and sauté the tofu and for about 6–7 minutes, or until golden-brown.    Add the garlic and pecans and sauté for about 1 minute.    Add the applesauce and cook for about 2 minutes.    Stir in the cilantro and remove from heat.    Transfer tofu into a plate and set aside    In the same skillet, heat the remaining oil over medium-high heat and cook the Brussels sprouts and bell peppers for about 5 minutes.    Stir in the tofu and remove from the heat.    Serve immediately.

**Nutrition Info:** Calories 238 Total Fat 17.8 g Saturated Fat 2 g Cholesterol 0 mg Sodium 26 mg Total Carbs 13.6 g Fiber 4.8 g Sugar 4.5 g Protein 11.8 g

## Grains Combo

Servings: 6    Cooking Time: 35 Minutes

**Ingredients:**
- ¾ cup amaranth
- 1 cup quinoa, rinsed
- ¼ cup wild rice
- 4¼ cups filtered water
- 2 teaspoons ground cumin
- ½ teaspoon paprika
- Salt, as required
- 1¼ cups boiled chickpeas
- 2 medium carrots, peeled and grated
- 1 garlic clove, minced
- Ground black pepper, as required

**Directions:**
In a large pan, add the amaranth, quinoa, wild rice, water and spices over medium-high heat and bring to a boil. Now, reduce the heat to medium-low and simmer, covered for about 20-25 minutes.    Stir in remaining ingredients and simmer for about 3-5 minutes.    Serve hot.    Meal Prep Tip: Transfer the grains mixture into a large bowl and set aside to cool. Divide the mixture into 6 containers evenly. Cover the containers and refrigerate for 1 day. Reheat in the microwave before serving.

**Nutrition Info:** Calories 365 Total Fat 5.6 g Saturated Fat 0.6 g Cholesterol 0 mg Total Carbs 64 g Sugar 5.8 g Fiber 12 g Sodium 58 mg Potassium 686 mg Protein 16.4 g

## Mixed Veggie Salad

Servings: 8

**Ingredients:**
- For Dressing:
- 1/3 cup olive oil
- ½ cup fresh lemon juice
- 1 tablespoon fresh ginger, grated
- 2 teaspoons mustard
- 4-6 drops liquid stevia
- ¼ teaspoon salt
- For Salad:
- 2 avocados, peeled, pitted and chopped
- 2 tablespoons fresh lemon juice
- 2 cups fresh baby spinach, torn
- 2 cups small broccoli florets
- 1 cup red cabbage, shredded
- 1 cup purple cabbage, shredded
- 2 large carrots, peeled and grated
- 1 small orange bell pepper, seeded and sliced into matchsticks
- 1 small yellow bell pepper, seeded and sliced into matchsticks
- ½ cup fresh parsley leaves, chopped
- 1 cup walnuts, chopped

**Directions:**

For dressing: in a food processor, add all ingredients and pulse until well combined. In a large bowl, add the avocado slices and drizzle with lemon juice. Add the remaining vegetables and mix. Place the dressing and toss to coat well. Serve immediately. Meal Prep Tip: Transfer dressing into a small jar and refrigerate for 1 day. In 8 containers, divide avocado and remaining vegetables. Refrigerate for 1 day. Before serving, drizzle each portion with dressing and serve.

**Nutrition Info:**Calories 314 Total Fat 28.1 g Saturated Fat 4 g Cholesterol 0 mg Total Carbs 14.1 g Sugar 4.3g Fiber 6.9 g Sodium 113 mg Potassium 642 mg Protein 6.8 g

## Zucchini With Tomatoes

Servings: 8     Cooking Time: 11 Minutes
**Ingredients:**
- 6 medium zucchinis, chopped roughly
- 1-pound cherry tomatoes
- 2 small onions, chopped roughly
- 2 tablespoons fresh basil, chopped
- 1 cup water
- 1 tablespoon olive oil
- 2 garlic cloves, minced
- Salt and ground black pepper, as required

**Directions:**
In the Instant Pot, place oil and press "Sauté". Now add the onion, garlic, ginger, and spices and cook for about 3-4 minutes. Add the zucchinis and tomatoes and cook for about 1-2 minutes. Press "Cancel" and stir in the remaining ingredients except basil. Close the lid and place the pressure valve to "Seal" position. Press "Manual" and cook under "High Pressure" for about 5 minutes. Press "Cancel" and allow a "Natural" release. Open the lid and transfer the vegetable mixture onto a serving platter. Garnish with basil and serve.

**Nutrition Info:**Calories: 57 Fats: 2.1g Carbohydrates: 9gSugar: 4.8gProteins: 2.5g Sodium: 39mg

## Tofu With Brussels Sprout

Servings: 4     Cooking Time: 15 Minutes
**Ingredients:**
- 1 tablespoon olive oil, divided
- 8 ounces extra-firm tofu, drained, pressed and cut into slices
- 2 garlic cloves, chopped
- 1/3 cup pecans, toasted and chopped
- 1 tablespoon unsweetened applesauce
- ¼ cup fresh cilantro, chopped
- ¾ pound Brussels sprouts, trimmed and cut into wide ribbons

**Directions:**
In a skillet, heat ½ tablespoon of the oil over medium heat and sauté the tofu and for about 6-7 minutes or until golden brown. Add the garlic and pecans and sauté for about 1 minute. Add the applesauce and cook for about 2 minutes. Stir in the cilantro and remove from heat. Transfer tofu into a plate and set aside In the same skillet, heat the remaining oil over medium-high heat and cook the Brussels sprouts for about 5 minutes. Stir in the tofu and remove from the heat. Serve

immediately. Meal Prep Tip: Remove the tofu mixture from heat and set aside to cool completely. In 4 containers, divide the tofu mixture evenly and refrigerate for about 2 days. Reheat in microwave before serving.

**Nutrition Info:**Calories 204 Total Fat 15.5 g Saturated Fat 1.8 g Cholesterol 0 mg Total Carbs 11.5 g Sugar 3 g Fiber 4.8 g Sodium 27 mg Potassium 468 mg Protein 9.9 g

## Baked Veggies Combo

Servings: 8     Cooking Time: 40 Minutes
**Ingredients:**
- 2 large zucchinis, sliced
- 1 large yellow squash, sliced
- 3 cups fresh broccoli florets
- 1 pound fresh asparagus, trimmed
- 2 garlic cloves, minced
- 1 tablespoon fresh rosemary, minced
- 1 tablespoon fresh thyme, minced
- ½ teaspoon ground cumin
- ½ teaspoon red pepper flakes, crushed
- ¼ teaspoon cayenne pepper
- 2 tablespoons olive oil
- Salt, as required

**Directions:**
Preheat the oven to 400 degrees F. Line 2 large baking sheets with aluminum foil. In a large bowl, add all ingredients and toss to coat well. Divide the vegetables mixture onto prepared baking sheets and spread in a single layer. Roast for about 35-40 minutes. Remove from oven and serve. Meal Prep Tip: Remove from oven and set the veggies aside to cool completely. Transfer the veggie mixture into 8 containers and refrigerate for 2-3 days. Reheat in microwave before serving.

**Nutrition Info:**Calories 77 Total Fat 4 g Saturated Fat 0.6 g Cholesterol 0 mg Total Carbs 9.4 g Sugar 3.8 g Fiber 3.8 g Sodium 45 mg Potassium 554 mg Protein 3.8 g

## Lentils Chili

Servings: 8     Cooking Time: 2 Hours 20 Minutes
**Ingredients:**
- 2 teaspoons olive oil
- 1 large onion, chopped
- 3 medium carrot, peeled and chopped
- 4 celery stalks, chopped
- 2 garlic cloves, minced
- 1 jalapeño pepper, seeded and chopped
- ½ tablespoon dried thyme, crushed
- 1 tablespoon chipotle chili powder
- ½ tablespoon cayenne pepper
- 1½ tablespoons ground coriander
- 1½ tablespoons ground cumin
- 1 teaspoon ground turmeric
- Ground black pepper, as required
- 1 tomato, chopped finely
- 1 pound lentils, rinsed
- 8 cups low-sodium vegetable broth
- 6 cups fresh spinach
- ½ cup fresh cilantro, chopped

**Directions:**
In a large pan, heat the oil over medium heat and sauté the onion, carrot and celery for about 5 minutes. Add the garlic, jalapeño pepper, thyme and spices and sauté for about 1 minute. Add the tomato paste, lentils and broth and bring to a boil. Now, reduce the heat to low and simmer for about 2 hours. Stir in the spinach and simmer for about 3-5 minutes. Stir in cilantro and remove from the heat. Serve hot. Meal Prep Tip: Transfer the chili into a large bowl and set aside to cool. Divide the chili into 8 containers evenly. Cover the containers and refrigerate for 1-2 days. Reheat in the microwave before serving.
**Nutrition Info:**Calories 259 Total Fat 2.3 g Saturated Fat 0.3 g Cholesterol 0 mg Total Carbs 41 g Sugar 3.6 g Fiber 19 g Sodium 118 mg Potassium 856 mg Protein 18.2 g

## Fried Tofu Hotpot

Servings: 2     Cooking Time: 15 Minutes
**Ingredients:**
● 0.5lb fried tofu
● 1lb chopped Chinese vegetable mix
● 1 cup low sodium vegetable broth
● 2tbsp 5 spice seasoning
● 1tbsp smoked paprika
**Directions:**
Mix all the ingredients in your Instant Pot. Cook on Stew for 15 minutes. Release the pressure naturally.
**Nutrition Info:**Calories: 320 Carbs: 11 Sugar: 3 Fat: 23 Protein: 47 GL: 6

## Seitan Curry

Servings: 2     Cooking Time: 20 Minutes
**Ingredients:**
● 0.5lb seitan
● 1 thinly sliced onion
● 1 cup chopped tomato
● 3tbsp curry paste
● 1tbsp oil or ghee
**Directions:**
Set the Instant Pot to saute and add the onion, oil, and curry paste. When the onion is soft, add the remaining ingredients and seal. Cook on Stew for 20 minutes. Release the pressure naturally.
**Nutrition Info:**Calories: 240 Carbs: 19 Sugar: 4 Fat: 10 Protein: 32 GL: 10

## Split Pea Stew

Servings: 2     Cooking Time: 35 Minutes
**Ingredients:**
● 1 cup dry split peas
● 1lb chopped vegetables
● 1 cup mushroom soup
● 2tbsp old bay seasoning
**Directions:**

Mix all the ingredients in your Instant Pot. Cook on Beans for 35 minutes. Release the pressure naturally.
**Nutrition Info:**Calories: 300 Carbs: 7 Sugar: 3 Fat: 2 Protein: 24 GL: 4

## Grilled Potatoes In A Packet

Servings: 6     Cooking Time: 35 Minutes
**Ingredients:**
● 1 ½ lb. potatoes, sliced into wedges
● 2 cloves garlic, sliced
● 2 tablespoons olive oil
● Salt and pepper to taste
● 1 teaspoon dried rosemary
**Directions:**
Preheat your grill. Create a packet using foil. Drizzle oil over the potatoes and season with salt, pepper and rosemary. Place potatoes inside the packet. Fold and seal. Grill for 15 minutes. Turn to the other side. Grill for 20 minutes. Remove from the grill and open cautiously. Serve while warm.
**Nutrition Info:**Calories 148 Total Fat 6 g Saturated Fat 1 g Cholesterol 0 mg Sodium 141 mg Total Carbohydrate 22 g Dietary Fiber 2 g Total Sugars 2 g Protein 3 g Potassium 626 mg

## Seitan Roast

Servings: 2     Cooking Time: 35 Minutes
**Ingredients:**
● 1lb seitan roulade
● 1lb chopped winter vegetables
● 1 cup low sodium vegetable broth
● 4tbsp roast rub
**Directions:**
Rub the roast rub into your roulade. Place the roulade and vegetables in your Instant Pot. Add the broth. Seal. Cook on Stew for 35 minutes. Release the pressure naturally.
**Nutrition Info:**Calories: 260 Carbs: 9 Sugar: 2 Fat: 2 Protein: 49 GL: 4

## Eggplant Curry

Servings: 2     Cooking Time: 20 Minutes
**Ingredients:**
● 2-3 cups chopped eggplant
● 1 thinly sliced onion
● 1 cup coconut milk
● 3tbsp curry paste
● 1tbsp oil or ghee
**Directions:**
Set the Instant Pot to saute and add the onion, oil, and curry paste. When the onion is soft, add the remaining ingredients and seal. Cook on Stew for 20 minutes. Release the pressure naturally.
**Nutrition Info:**Calories: 350 Carbs: 15 Sugar: 3 Fat: 25 Protein: 11 GL: 10

# Soup And Stew Recipes

## Irish Stew

Servings: 2      Cooking Time: 35 Minutes

**Ingredients:**
- 1.5lb diced lamb shoulder
- 1lb chopped vegetables
- 1 cup low sodium beef broth
- 3 minced onions
- 1tbsp ghee

**Directions:**

Mix all the ingredients in your Instant Pot.      Cook on Stew for 35 minutes.      Release the pressure naturally.

**Nutrition Info:**Calories: 330; Carbs: 9; Sugar: 2; Fat: 12; Protein: 49; GL: 3

## Vegetarian Split Pea Soup In A Crock Pot

Servings: 8      Cooking Time: 10 Minutes

**Ingredients:**
- 2 chopped ribs celery
- 2 cubes low-sodium bouillon
- 8 c. water
- 2 c. uncooked green split peas
- 3 bay leaves
- 2 carrots
- 2 chopped potatoes
- Pepper and salt

**Directions:**

In your Crock-Pot, put the bouillon cubes, split peas, and water. Stir a bit to break up the bouillon cubes.      Next, add the chopped potatoes, celery, and carrots followed with bay leaves.      Stir to combine well.      Cover and cook for at least 4 hours on your Crock-Pot's low setting or until the green split peas are soft.      Add a bit salt and pepper as needed.      Before serving, remove the bay leaves and enjoy.

**Nutrition Info:**Calories: 149, Fat:1 g, Carbs:30 g, Protein:7 g, Sugars:3 g, Sodium:732 mg

## Thai Peanut, Carrot, & Shrimp Soup

Servings: 4      Cooking Time: 10 Minutes

**Ingredients:**
- 3 garlic cloves, minced
- ½ onion, sliced
- 1 tablespoon Thai red curry paste
- 1 tablespoon coconut oil
- fresh cilantro, minced, for garnish
- ½ pound shrimp, peeled and deveined
- ½ cup unsweetened plain almond milk
- 4 cups of low-sodium vegetable broth
- ½ cup whole unsalted peanuts
- 2 cups carrots, chopped

**Directions:**

In a pan, heat your oil over medium-high heat until shimmering.      Add your curry paste to the pan and cook continually stirring for about 1 minute. Add the garlic, onion, and carrots, along with peanuts to the pan. Continue cooking for 3 minutes or until your onion begins to soften.      Add your broth and bring to a boil. Reduce heat to a low setting and simmer for 6 minutes or until carrots are tender.      Use your immersion blender to puree your soup until smooth and return to pot. With heat setting on low, add the almond milk and stir to combine. Add your shrimp to the pot and cook for 3 minutes or until cooked.      Garnish soup with cilantro, then serve and enjoy!

**Nutrition Info:**Carbs per serving: 17g

## Ham Asparagus Soup

Servings: 3-4      Cooking Time: 55 Min.

**Ingredients:**
- 5 crushed garlic cloves
- 1 cup chopped ham
- 4 cups (preferably homemade) chicken broth
- 2 pounds trimmed and halved asparagus spears
- 2 tablespoons butter
- 1 chopped yellow onion
- ½ teaspoon dried thyme
- Salt and freshly (finely ground) black pepper, as per taste preference

**Directions:**

Arrange Instant Pot over a dry platform in your kitchen. Open its top lid and switch it on.      Find and press "SAUTE" cooking function; add the butter in it and allow it to heat.      In the pot, add the onions; cook (while stirring) until turns translucent and softened for around 4-5 minutes.      Add the garlic, ham bone and broth; stir, and cook for about 2-3 minutes.      Add the other ingredients; gently stir to mix well.      Close the lid to create a locked chamber; make sure that safety valve is in locking position.      Find and press "SOUP" cooking function; timer to 45 minutes with default "HIGH" pressure mode.      Allow the pressure to build to cook the ingredients.      After cooking time is over press "CANCEL" setting. Find and press "QPR" cooking function. This setting is for quick release of inside pressure.      Slowly open the lid, add the mix in a blender or processor.      Blend or process to make a smooth mix. Place the mix in serving bowls and enjoy the keto.

**Nutrition Info:**Calories - 146 Fat: 7g Saturated Fat: 3g Trans Fat: 0g Carbohydrates: 5g Fiber: 4g Sodium: 262mg Protein: 10g

## Cabbage Soup

Servings: 2      Cooking Time: 35 Minutes

**Ingredients:**
- 1lb shredded cabbage
- 1 cup low sodium vegetable broth
- 1 shredded onion
- 2tbsp mixed herbs
- 1tbsp black pepper

**Directions:**

Mix all the ingredients in your Instant Pot.      Cook on Stew for 35 minutes.      Release the pressure naturally.

**Nutrition Info:**Calories: 60; Carbs: 2; Sugar: 0; Fat: 2; Protein: 4; GL: 1

## Chickpea Soup

Servings: 2     Cooking Time: 35 Minutes
**Ingredients:**
- 1lb cooked chickpeas
- 1lb chopped vegetables
- 1 cup low sodium vegetable broth
- 2tbsp mixed herbs

**Directions:**
Mix all the ingredients in your Instant Pot.     Cook on Stew for 35 minutes.     Release the pressure naturally.
**Nutrition Info:**Calories: 310; Carbs: 20; Sugar: 3; Fat: 5; Protein: 27; GL: 5

## Meatball Stew

Servings: 2     Cooking Time: 25 Minutes
**Ingredients:**
- 1lb sausage meat
- 2 cups chopped tomato
- 1 cup chopped vegetables
- 2tbsp Italian seasonings
- 1tbsp vegetable oil

**Directions:**
Roll the sausage into meatballs.     Put the Instant Pot on Sauté and fry the meatballs in the oil until brown.     Mix all the ingredients in your Instant Pot.     Cook on Stew for 25 minutes.     Release the pressure naturally.
**Nutrition Info:**Calories: 300; Carbs: 4; Sugar: 1; Fat: 12; Protein: 40; GL: 2

## Squash Soup

Servings: 6     Cooking Time: 8 Hours
**Ingredients:**
- 2 lb butternut squash, peeled, chopped into chunks
- 1 tsp ginger, minced
- 1/4 tsp cinnamon
- 1 Tbsp curry powder
- 2 bay leaves
- 1 tsp black pepper
- 1/2 cup heavy cream
- 2 cups chicken stock
- 1 Tbsp garlic, minced
- 2 carrots, cut into chunks
- 2 apples, peeled, cored and diced
- 1 large onion, diced
- 1 tsp salt

**Directions:**
Spray a crock pot inside with cooking spray.     Add all ingredients except cream to the crock pot and stir well.     Cover and cook on low for 8 hours.     Purée the soup using an immersion blender until smooth and creamy.     Stir in heavy cream and season soup with pepper and salt.     Serve and enjoy.
**Nutrition Info:**Calories 170 Fat 4.4 g Carbohydrates 34.4 g Sugar 13.4g Protein 2.9 g Cholesterol 14 mg

## French Onion Soup

Servings: 2     Cooking Time: 35 Minutes
**Ingredients:**
- 6 onions, chopped finely
- 2 cups vegetable broth
- 2tbsp oil
- 2tbsp Gruyere

**Directions:**
Place the oil in your Instant Pot and cook the onions on Sauté until soft and brown.     Mix all the ingredients in your Instant Pot.     Cook on Stew for 35 minutes.     Release the pressure naturally.
**Nutrition Info:**Calories: 110; Carbs: 8; Sugar: 3; Fat: 10; Protein: 3; GL: 4

## Cherry Stew

Servings: 6     Cooking Time: 10 Minutes
**Ingredients:**
- 2 c. water
- ½ c. powered cocoa
- ¼ c. coconut sugar
- 1 lb. pitted cherries

**Directions:**
In a pan, combine the cherries with all the water, sugar plus the hot chocolate mix, stir, cook over medium heat for ten minutes, divide into bowls and serve cold. Enjoy!
**Nutrition Info:**Calories: 207, Fat:1 g, Carbs:8 g, Protein:6 g, Sugars:27 g, Sodium:19 mg

## Curried Carrot Soup

Servings: 6     Cooking Time: 5 Minutes
**Ingredients:**
- 2 celery stalks, chopped
- 1 small onion, chopped
- 1 tablespoon extra-virgin olive oil
- 1 tablespoon fresh cilantro, chopped
- ¼ teaspoon freshly ground black pepper
- 1 cup of canned coconut milk
- ¼ teaspoon salt
- 4 cups of low-sodium vegetable broth
- 6 medium carrots, roughly chopped
- 1 teaspoon fresh ginger, minced
- 1 teaspoon ground cumin
- 1 ½ teaspoon curry powder

**Directions:**
Heat your Instant Pot to high setting and add the olive oil. Sauté your celery and onion for 3 minutes. Add the curry powder, ginger, and cumin to the pot and cook for about 30 seconds.     Add the carrots, vegetable broth, and salt to your pot. Close pot and seal and set on high for 5 minutes. Allow the pressure to release naturally.     Pure your soup in batches in a blender jar and transfer back into the pot.     Stir in the coconut milk along with pepper and heat through. Top soup with cilantro, then serve and enjoy!
**Nutrition Info:**Carbs per serving: 13g

## Vegan Cream Soup With Avocado & Zucchini

Servings: 2     Cooking Time: 20 Minutes
**Ingredients:**
- 3 tsp vegetable oil
- 1 leek, chopped
- 1 rutabaga, sliced

- 3 cups zucchinis, chopped
- 1 avocado, chopped
- Salt and black pepper to taste
- 4 cups vegetable broth
- 2 tbsp fresh mint, chopped

**Directions:**

In a pot, sauté leek, zucchini, and rutabaga in warm oil for about 7-10 minutes. Season with black pepper and salt. Pour in broth and bring to a boil. Lower the heat and simmer for 20 minutes. Lift from the heat. In batches, add the soup and avocado to a blender. Blend until creamy and smooth. Serve in bowls topped with fresh mint.

**Nutrition Info:**Calories 378 Fat: 24.5g, Net Carbs: 9.3g, Protein: 8.2g

## Kebab Stew

Servings: 2      Cooking Time: 35 Minutes

**Ingredients:**
- 1lb cubed, seasoned kebab meat
- 1lb cooked chickpeas
- 1 cup low sodium vegetable broth
- 1tbsp black pepper

**Directions:**

Mix all the ingredients in your Instant Pot.      Cook on Stew for 35 minutes.      Release the pressure naturally.

**Nutrition Info:**Calories: 290; Carbs: 22; Sugar: 4; Fat: 10; Protein: 34; GL: 6

## Meatless Ball Soup

Servings: 2      Cooking Time: 15 Minutes

**Ingredients:**
- 1lb minced tofu
- 0.5lb chopped vegetables
- 2 cups low sodium vegetable broth
- 1tbsp almond flour
- salt and pepper

**Directions:**

Mix the tofu, flour, salt and pepper.      Form the meatballs.      Place all the ingredients in your Instant Pot. Cook on Stew for 15 minutes.      Release the pressure naturally.

**Nutrition Info:**Calories: 240; Carbs: 9; Sugar: 3; Fat: 10; Protein: 35; GL: 5

## Tofu Soup

Servings: 8      Cooking Time: 10 Minutes

**Ingredients:**
- 1 lb. cubed extra-firm tofu
- 3 diced medium carrots
- 8 c. low-sodium vegetable broth
- ½ tsp. freshly ground white pepper
- 8 minced garlic cloves
- 6 sliced and divided scallions
- 4 oz. sliced mushrooms
- 1-inch minced fresh ginger piece

**Directions:**

Pour the broth into a stockpot. Add all of the ingredients except for the tofu and last 2 scallions. Bring to a boil over high heat.      Once boiling, add the tofu. Reduce heat to

low, cover, and simmer for 5 minutes.      Remove from heat, ladle soup into bowls, and garnish with the remaining sliced scallions. Serve immediately.

**Nutrition Info:**Calories: 91, Fat:3 g, Carbs:8 g, Protein:6 g, Sugars:4 g, Sodium:900 mg

## Chicken Zoodle Soup

Servings: 2      Cooking Time: 35 Minutes

**Ingredients:**
- 1lb chopped cooked chicken
- 1lb spiralized zucchini
- 1 cup low sodium chicken soup
- 1 cup diced vegetables

**Directions:**

Mix all the ingredients except the zucchini in your Instant Pot.      Cook on Stew for 35 minutes.      Release the pressure naturally.      Stir in the zucchini and allow to heat thoroughly.

**Nutrition Info:**Calories: 250; Carbs: 5; Sugar: 0; Fat: 10; Protein: 40; GL: 1

## Cheese Cream Soup With Chicken & Cilantro

Servings: 4      Cooking Time: 10 Minutes

**Ingredients:**
- 1 carrot, chopped
- 1 onion, chopped
- 2 cups cooked and shredded chicken
- 3 tbsp butter
- 4 cups chicken broth
- 2 tbsp cilantro, chopped
- 1/3 cup buffalo sauce
- ½ cup cream cheese
- Salt and black pepper, to taste

**Directions:**

In a skillet over medium heat, warm butter and sauté carrot and onion until tender, about 5 minutes.      Add to a food processor and blend with buffalo sauce and cream cheese, until smooth. Transfer to a pot, add chicken broth and heat until hot but do not bring to a boil. Stir in chicken, salt, pepper and cook until heated through. When ready, remove to soup bowls and serve garnished with cilantro.

**Nutrition Info:**Calories 487, Fat: 41g, Net Carbs: 7.2g, Protein: 16.3g

## Spicy Pepper Soup

Servings: 2      Cooking Time: 15 Minutes

**Ingredients:**
- 1lb chopped mixed sweet peppers
- 1 cup low sodium vegetable broth
- 3tbsp chopped chili peppers
- 1tbsp black pepper

**Directions:**

Mix all the ingredients in your Instant Pot.      Cook on Stew for 15 minutes.      Release the pressure naturally. Blend.

**Nutrition Info:**Calories: 100; Carbs: 11; Sugar: 4; Fat: 2; Protein: 3; GL: 6

## Awesome Chicken Enchilada Soup

Servings: 4    Cooking Time: 30 Minutes

**Ingredients:**
- 2 tbsp coconut oil
- 1 lb boneless, skinless chicken thighs
- ¾ cup red enchilada sauce, sugar-free
- ¼ cup water
- ¼ cup onion, chopped
- 3 oz canned diced green chilis
- 1 avocado, sliced
- 1 cup cheddar cheese, shredded
- ¼ cup pickled jalapeños, chopped
- ½ cup sour cream
- 1 tomato, diced

**Directions:**
Put a large pan over medium heat. Add coconut oil and warm. Place in the chicken and cook until browned on the outside. Stir in onion, chillis, water, and enchilada sauce, then close with a lid.    Allow simmering for 20 minutes until the chicken is cooked through.    Spoon the soup on a serving bowl and top with the sauce, cheese, sour cream, tomato, and avocado.

**Nutrition Info:**Calories: 643, Fat: 44.2g, Net Carbs: 9.7g, Protein: 45.8g

## Zucchini-basil Soup

Servings: 5    Cooking Time: 10 Minutes

**Ingredients:**
- 1/3 c. packed basil leaves
- ¾ c. chopped onion
- ¼ c. olive oil
- 2 lbs. trimmed and sliced zucchini
- 2 chopped garlic cloves
- 4 c. divided water

**Directions:**
Peel and julienne the skin from half of zucchini; toss with 1/2 teaspoon salt and drain in a sieve until wilted, at least 20 minutes. Coarsely chop remaining zucchini.    Cook onion and garlic in oil in a saucepan over medium-low heat, stirring occasionally, until onions are translucent. Add chopped zucchini and 1 teaspoon salt and cook, stirring occasionally.    Add 3 cups water and simmer with the lid ajar until tender. Pour the soup in a blender and purée soup with basil.    Bring remaining cup water to a boil in a small saucepan and blanch julienned zucchini. Drain.    Top soup with julienned zucchini. Season soup with salt and pepper and serve.

**Nutrition Info:**Calories: 169.3, Fat:13.7 g, Carbs:12 g, Protein:2 g,Sugars:3.8 g, Sodium:8 mg

## Sweet And Sour Soup

Servings: 2    Cooking Time: 35 Minutes

**Ingredients:**
- 1lb cubed chicken breast
- 1lb chopped vegetables
- 1 cup low carb sweet and sour sauce
- 0.5 cup diabetic marmalade

**Directions:**
Mix all the ingredients in your Instant Pot.    Cook on Stew for 35 minutes.    Release the pressure naturally.

**Nutrition Info:**Calories: 305; Carbs: 4; Sugar: 1.2; Fat: 12; Protein: 40; GL: 2

## Curried Shrimp & Green Bean Soup

Servings: 4    Cooking Time: 10 Minutes

**Ingredients:**
- 1 onion, chopped
- 2 tbsp red curry paste
- 2 tbsp butter
- 1-pound jumbo shrimp, peeled and deveined
- 2 tsp ginger-garlic puree
- 1 cup coconut milk
- Salt and chili pepper to taste
- 1 bunch green beans, halved
- 1 tbsp cilantro, chopped

**Directions:**
Add the shrimp to melted butter in a saucepan over medium heat, season with salt and pepper, and cook until they are opaque, 2 to 3 minutes. Remove to a plate. Add in the ginger-garlic puree, onion, and red curry paste and sauté for 2 minutes until fragrant.    Stir in the coconut milk; add the shrimp, salt, chili pepper, and green beans. Cook for 4 minutes. Reduce the heat to a simmer and cook an additional 3 minutes, occasionally stirring. Adjust taste with salt, fetch soup into serving bowls, and serve sprinkled with cilantro.

**Nutrition Info:**Calories 351, Fat 32.4g, Net Carbs 3.2g, Protein 7.7g

## Beef Borscht Soup

Servings: 8    Cooking Time: 30 Minutes

**Ingredients:**
- 2 lbs ground beef
- 3 beets, peeled and diced
- 2 large carrots, diced
- 3 stalks of celery, diced
- 1 onion, diced
- 2 cloves garlic, diced
- 3 cups shredded cabbage
- 6 cups beef stock
- ½ tbsp thyme
- 1 bay leaf
- Salt and ground black pepper to taste

**Directions:**
Preheat the Instant Pot by selecting SAUTÉ.    Add the ground beef and cook, stirring, for 5 minutes, until browned.    Combine all the rest ingredients in the Instant Pot and stir to mix. Close and lock the lid. Press the CANCEL button to stop the SAUTE function, then select the MANUAL setting and set the cooking time for 15 minutes at HIGH pressure.    Once timer goes off, allow to Naturally Release for 10 minutes, then release any remaining pressure manually. Uncover the pot.    Let the dish sit for 5-10 minutes and serve.

**Nutrition Info:**Calories 301 Fat 27.2 g Carbohydrates 13.6 g Sugar 6 g Protein 3 g Cholesterol 33 mg

## Broccoli & Spinach Soup

Servings: 4    Cooking Time: 20 Minutes

**Ingredients:**

- 2 tbsp butter
- 1 onion, chopped
- 1 garlic clove, minced
- 2 heads broccoli, cut in florets
- 2 stalks celery, chopped
- 4 cups vegetable broth
- 1 cup baby spinach
- Salt and black pepper to taste
- 1 tbsp basil, chopped
- Parmesan cheese, shaved to serve

**Directions:**
Melt the butter in a saucepan over medium heat. Sauté the garlic and onion for 3 minutes until softened. Mix in the broccoli and celery, and cook for 4 minutes until slightly tender. Pour in the broth, bring to a boil, then reduce the heat to medium-low and simmer covered for about 5 minutes. Drop in the spinach to wilt, adjust the seasonings, and cook for 4 minutes. Ladle soup into serving bowls. Serve with a sprinkle of grated Parmesan cheese and chopped basil.
**Nutrition Info:** Calories 123 Fat 11g Net Carbs 3.2g Protein 1.8g

## Vegetable Chicken Soup

Servings: 6     Cooking Time: 6 Hours
**Ingredients:**
- 4 cups chicken, boneless, skinless, cooked and diced
- 4 tsp garlic, minced
- 2/3 cups onion, diced
- 1 1/2 cups carrot, diced
- 6 cups chicken stock
- 2 Tbsp lime juice
- 1/4 cup jalapeño pepper, diced
- 1/2 cup tomatoes, diced
- 1/2 cup fresh cilantro, chopped
- 1 tsp chili powder
- 1 Tbsp cumin
- 1 3/4 cups tomato juice
- 2 tsp sea salt

**Directions:**
Add all ingredients to a crock pot and stir well. Cover and cook on low for 6 hours. Stir well and serve.
**Nutrition Info:** Calories 192 Fat 3.8 g Carbohydrates 9.8 g Sugar 5.7 g Protein 29.2 g Cholesterol 72 mg

## Beef Barley Soup

Servings: 8     Cooking Time: 30 Minutes
**Ingredients:**
- 2 tbsp olive oil
- 2 lbs beef chuck roast, cut into 1½ inch steaks
- Salt and ground black pepper to taste
- 2 onions, chopped
- 4 cloves of garlic, sliced
- 4 large carrots, chopped
- 1 stalk of celery, chopped
- 1 cup pearl barley, rinsed
- 1 bay leaf
- 8 cups chicken stock
- 1 tbsp fish sauce

**Directions:**

Select the SAUTÉ setting on the Instant Pot and heat the oil. Sprinkle the beef with salt and pepper. Put in the pot and brown for about 5 minutes. Turn and brown the other side. Remove the meat from the pot. Add the onion, garlic, carrots, and celery. Stir and sauté for 6 minutes. Return the beef to the pot. Add the pearl barley, bay leaf, chicken stock and fish sauce. Stir well. Close and lock the lid. Press the CANCEL button to reset the cooking program, then press the MANUAL button and set the cooking time for 30 minutes at HIGH pressure. Once cooking is complete, let the pressure Release Naturally for 15 minutes. Release any remaining steam manually. Uncover the pot. Remove cloves garlic, large vegetable chunks and bay leaf. Taste for seasoning and add more salt if needed.
**Nutrition Info:** Calories 200 Fat 27.2 g Carbohydrates 13.6 g Sugar 2 g Protein 4.4 g Cholesterol 32 mg

## Sirloin Carrot Soup

Servings: 6     Cooking Time: 10 Minutes
**Ingredients:**
- 1 lb. chopped carrots and celery mix
- 32 oz. low-sodium beef stock
- 1/3 c. whole-wheat flour
- 1 lb. ground beef sirloin
- 1 tbsp. olive oil
- 1 chopped yellow onion

**Directions:**
Heat up the olive oil in a saucepan over medium-high flame; add the beef and the flour. Stir well and cook to brown for 4-5 minutes. Add the celery, onion, carrots, and stock; stir and bring to a simmer. Turn down the heat to low and cook for 12-15 minutes. Serve warm.
**Nutrition Info:** Calories: 140, Fat: 4.5 g, Carbs: 16 g, Protein: 9 g, Sugars: 3 g, Sodium:670 mg

## Mexican Chicken Soup

Servings: 6     Cooking Time: 4 Hours
**Ingredients:**
- 1 1/2 lb chicken thighs, skinless and boneless
- 14 oz chicken stock
- 14 oz salsa
- 8 oz Monterey Jack cheese, shredded

**Directions:**
Place chicken into a crock pot. Pour remaining ingredients over the chicken. Cover and cook on high for 4 hours. Remove chicken from crock pot and shred using forks. Return shredded chicken to the crock pot and stir well. Serve and enjoy.
**Nutrition Info:** Calories 371 Fat 19.5 g Carbohydrates 5.7 g Sugar 2.2 g Protein 42.1 g Cholesterol 135 mg

## Mushroom Cream Soup With Herbs

Servings: 4     Cooking Time: 15 Minutes
**Ingredients:**
- 1 onion, chopped
- ½ cup crème fraiche
- ¼ cup butter
- 12 oz white mushrooms, chopped
- 1 tsp thyme leaves, chopped

- 1 tsp parsley leaves, chopped
- 1 tsp cilantro leaves, chopped
- 2 garlic cloves, minced
- 4 cups vegetable broth
- Salt and black pepper, to taste

**Directions:**
Add butter, onion and garlic to a large pot over high heat and cook for 3 minutes until tender. Add mushrooms, salt and pepper, and cook for 10 minutes. Pour in the broth and bring to a boil.   Reduce the heat and simmer for 10 minutes. Puree the soup with a hand blender until smooth. Stir in crème fraiche. Garnish with herbs before serving.

**Nutrition Info:**Calories 213 Fat: 18g Net Carbs: 4.1g Protein: 3.1g

## Beef & Mushroom Barley Soup

Servings: 6    Cooking Time: 1 Hour And 20 Minutes
**Ingredients:**
- ½ cup of pearl barley
- 1 cup of water
- 4 cups of low-sodium beef broth
- ½ teaspoon thyme, dried
- 6 garlic cloves, minced
- 3 celery stalks, chopped
- 1 onion, chopped
- 2 carrots, chopped
- 8-ounces of mushrooms, sliced
- 1 tablespoon extra-virgin olive oil
- ¼ teaspoon freshly ground black pepper
- 1 lb. Of beef stew meat, cubed

**Directions:**
Season your meat with salt and pepper.   Heat the oil in an Instant Pot over high heat. Add the beef and brown, then remove meat and set aside.   Add your mushrooms to the pot and cook for about 1 to 2 minutes or until they begin to soften. Remove the mushrooms from pot and set them aside along with the meat.   Add your carrots, celery, and onions into the pot. Sauté vegetables for about 4 minutes or until they begin to soften. Add your garlic into pot and cook until fragrant. Place the meat and mushrooms back into the pot, then add the beef broth, thyme, and water. Set your pot pressure to high and cook for 15 minutes. Allow the pressure to release naturally.   Open your Instant Pot and add the barley. Use the slow cooker function on the pot, with the lid having vent open, then continue cooking for an additional hour or until your barley is cooked and tender. Serve and enjoy!

**Nutrition Info:**Carbs per serving: 19g

## Spicy Chicken Pepper Stew

Servings: 6    Cooking Time: 6 Hours
**Ingredients:**
- 3 chicken breasts, skinless and boneless, cut into small pieces
- 1 tsp garlic, minced
- 1 tsp ground ginger
- 2 tsp olive oil
- 2 tsp soy sauce
- 1 Tbsp fresh lemon juice

- 1/2 cup green onions, sliced
- 1 Tbsp crushed red pepper
- 8 oz chicken stock
- 1 bell pepper, chopped
- 1 green chili pepper, sliced
- 2 jalapeño peppers, sliced
- 1/2 tsp black pepper
- 1/4 tsp sea salt

**Directions:**
Add all ingredients to a large mixing bowl and mix well. Place in the refrigerator overnight.   Pour marinated chicken mixture into a crock pot.   Cover and cook on low for 6 hours.   Stir well and serve.

**Nutrition Info:**Calories 171 Fat 7.4 g Carbohydrates 3.7 g Sugar 1.7 g Protein 22 g Cholesterol 65 mg

## Cream Pepper Stew

Servings: 4    Cooking Time: 10 Min.
**Ingredients:**
- 1 (preferably medium size) celery stalk, chopped
- 1 (preferably medium size) yellow bell pepper, chopped
- 1 (preferably medium size) green bell pepper, chopped
- 2 large red bell peppers, chopped
- 1 small red onion, chopped
- 2 tablespoons butter
- 1/2 cup cream cheese, full-fat
- 1/4 teaspoon dried thyme, (finely ground)
- 1/2 teaspoon black pepper, (finely ground)
- 1 teaspoon dried parsley, (finely ground)
- 1 teaspoon salt
- 2 cups vegetable stock
- 1 cup heavy cream

**Directions:**
Arrange Instant Pot over a dry platform in your kitchen. Open its top lid and switch it on.   Find and press "SAUTE" cooking function; add the butter in it and allow it to heat.   In the pot, add the onions, bell pepper, and celery; cook (while stirring) until turns translucent and softened for around 3-4 minutes.   Pour in the vegetable stock and heavy cream — season with salt, pepper, parsley, and thyme.   Close the lid to create a locked chamber; make sure that safety valve is in locking position.   Find and press "MANUAL" cooking function; timer to 6 minutes with default "HIGH" pressure mode.   Allow the pressure to build to cook the ingredients.   After cooking time is over press "CANCEL" setting. Find and press "QPR" cooking function. This setting is for quick release of inside pressure.   Slowly open the lid, mix in the cream; take out the cooked in serving plates or serving bowls, and enjoy the keto .

**Nutrition Info:**Calories - 286 Fat: 27g Saturated Fat: 6g Trans Fat: 0g Carbohydrates: 9g Fiber: 3g Sodium: 523mg Protein: 5g

## Easy Beef Mushroom Stew

Servings: 8    Cooking Time: 8 Hours
**Ingredients:**
- 2 lb stewing beef, cubed

- 1 packet dry onion soup mix
- 4 oz can mushrooms, sliced
- 14 oz can cream of mushroom soup
- 1/2 cup water
- 1/4 tsp black pepper
- 1/2 tsp salt

**Directions:**
Spray a crock pot inside with cooking spray. Add all ingredients into the crock pot and stir well. Cover and cook on low for 8 hours. Stir well and serve.
**Nutrition Info:** Calories 237 Fat 8.5 g Carbohydrates 2.7 g Sugar 0.4 g Protein 35.1 g Cholesterol 101 mg

## Summer Squash Soup With Crispy Chickpeas

Servings: 4    Cooking Time: 20 Minutes
**Ingredients:**
- ¼ teaspoon smoked paprika
- 1 teaspoon extra-virgin olive oil, plus one tablespoon
- 1 (15-ounce) can low-sodium chickpeas, drained and rinsed
- 2 tablespoons plain low-fat Greek yogurt
- freshly ground black pepper
- 3 garlic cloves, minced
- ½ onion, diced
- 3 cups of low-sodium vegetable broth
- 3 medium zucchinis, coarsely chopped
- pinch of sea salt, plus ½ teaspoon

**Directions:**
Preheat your oven to 425° Fahrenheit. Line a baking sheet with some parchment paper. In a mixing bowl, toss your chickpeas with one teaspoon of olive oil, the smoked paprika, and a pinch of sea salt. Transfer your mixture to the baking sheet, then roast until crispy for about 20 minutes, stirring once. Set aside. In a pot, heat the remaining 1 tablespoon of oil over medium heat. Add your zucchini, onion, broth, and garlic to the pot and bring to a boil. Lower the heat to simmer, then cook until the onion and zucchini are tender, for about 20 minutes. In a blender jar, puree your soup, then return it to the pot. Add the yogurt, and the remaining ½ teaspoon of sea salt, and pepper, then stir well. Serve topped with roasted chickpeas and enjoy!
**Nutrition Info:** Carbs per serving: 24g

## Healthy Chicken Kale Soup

Servings: 6    Cooking Time: 6 Hours 15 Minutes
**Ingredients:**
- 2 lb chicken breasts, skinless and boneless
- 1/4 cup fresh lemon juice
- 5 oz baby kale
- 32 oz chicken stock
- 1/2 cup olive oil
- 1 large onion, sliced
- 14 oz chicken broth
- 1 Tbsp extra-virgin olive oil
- Salt

**Directions:**
Heat the extra-virgin olive oil in a pan over medium heat. Season chicken with salt and place in the hot pan. Cover pan and cook chicken for 15 minutes. Remove chicken from the pan and shred it using forks. Add shredded chicken to a crock pot. Add sliced onion, olive oil, and broth to a blender and blend until combined. Pour blended mixture into the crock pot. Add remaining ingredients to the crock pot and stir well. Cover and cook on low for 6 hours. Stir well and serve.
**Nutrition Info:** Calories 493 Fat 31.3 g Carbohydrates 5.8 g Sugar 1.9 g Protein 46.7 g Cholesterol 135 mg

## Easy Beef Stew

Servings: 6    Cooking Time: 5 Minutes
**Ingredients:**
- 1 shredded green cabbage head
- 4 chopped carrots
- 2 ½ lbs. non-fat beef brisket
- 3 chopped garlic cloves
- Black pepper
- 2 bay leaves
- 4 c. low-sodium beef stock

**Directions:**
Put the beef brisket in a pot, add stock, pepper, garlic and bay leaves, provide your simmer over medium heat and cook for an hour. Add carrots and cabbage, stir, cook for a half-hour more, divide into bowls and serve for lunch. Enjoy!
**Nutrition Info:** Calories: 271, Fat:8 g, Carbs:16 g, Protein:9 g, Sugars:3.4 g, Sodium:760 mg

## Chicken Bacon Soup

Servings: 4    Cooking Time: 40 Minutes
**Ingredients:**
- 6 boneless, skinless chicken thighs, make cubes
- ½ cup chopped celery
- 4 minced garlic cloves
- 6-ounce mushrooms, sliced
- ½ cup chopped onion
- 8-ounce softened cream cheese
- ¼ cup softened butter
- 1 teaspoon dried thyme
- Salt and (finely ground) black pepper, as per taste preference
- 2 cups chopped spinach
- 8 ounces cooked bacon slices, chopped
- 3 cups (preferably homemade) chicken broth
- 1 cup heavy cream

**Directions:**
Arrange Instant Pot over a dry platform in your kitchen. Open its top lid and switch it on. Add the ingredients except for the cream, spinach, and bacon; gently stir to mix well. Close the lid to create a locked chamber; make sure that safety valve is in locking position. Find and press "SOUP" cooking function; timer to 30 minutes with default "HIGH" pressure mode. Allow the pressure to build to cook the ingredients. After cooking time is over press "CANCEL" setting. Find and press "NPR" cooking function. This setting is for the natural release of inside pressure and it takes around 10 minutes to slowly release pressure. Slowly open the lid, stir in cream and spinach. Take out the cooked in serving plates or serving bowls and enjoy the keto. Top with the bacon.

**Nutrition Info:**Calories - 456 Fat: 38g Saturated Fat: 13g Trans Fat: 0g Carbohydrates: 7g Fiber: 1g Sodium: 742mg Protein: 23g

## Rhubarb Stew

Servings: 3    Cooking Time: 10 Minutes
**Ingredients:**
- 1 tsp. grated lemon zest
- 1 ½ c. coconut sugar
- Juice of 1 lemon
- 1 ½ c. water
- 4 ½ c. roughly chopped rhubarbs

**Directions:**
In a pan, combine the rhubarb while using water, fresh lemon juice, lemon zest and coconut sugar, toss, bring using a simmer over medium heat, cook for 5 minutes, and divide into bowls and serve cold.    Enjoy!
**Nutrition Info:**Calories: 108, Fat:1 g, Carbs:8 g, Protein:5 g, Sugars:2 g, Sodium:0 mg

## Buffalo Chicken Soup

Servings: 8    Cooking Time: 30 Minutes
**Ingredients:**
- 2 chicken breasts, boneless, skinless, frozen or fresh
- 1 clove garlic, chopped
- ¼ cup onion, diced
- ½ cup celery, diced
- 2 tbsp butter
- 1 tbsp ranch dressing mix
- 3 cups chicken broth
- 1/3 cup hot sauce
- 2 cups cheddar cheese, shredded
- 1 cup heavy cream

**Directions:**
In the Instant Pot, combine the chicken breasts, garlic, onion, celery, butter, ranch dressing mix, broth, and hot sauce.    Close and lock the lid. Select MANUAL and cook at HIGH pressure for 10 minutes.    Once cooking is complete, let the pressure Release Naturally for 10 minutes. Release any remaining steam manually. Uncover the pot.    Transfer the chicken to a plate and shred the meat.    Return to the pot.    Add the cheese and heavy cream. Stir well. Let sit for 5 minutes and serve.
**Nutrition Info:**Calories 303 Fat 27.5 g Carbohydrates 13.8 g Sugar 5 g Protein 4.g Cholesterol 33 mg

## Chinese Tofu Soup

Servings: 2    Cooking Time: 10 Minutes
**Ingredients:**
- 2 cups chicken stock
- 1 tbsp soy sauce, sugar-free
- 2 spring onions, sliced
- 1 tsp sesame oil, softened
- 2 eggs, beaten
- 1-inch piece ginger, grated
- Salt and black ground, to taste
- ½ pound extra-firm tofu, cubed
- A handful of fresh cilantro, chopped

**Directions:**

Boil in a pan over medium heat, soy sauce, chicken stock and sesame oil. Place in eggs as you whisk to incorporate completely. Change heat to low and add salt, spring onions, black pepper and ginger; cook for 5 minutes. Place in tofu and simmer for 1 to 2 minutes.    Divide into soup bowls and serve sprinkled with fresh cilantro.
**Nutrition Info:**Calories 163; Fat: 10g, Net Carbs: 2.4g, Protein: 14.5g

## Healthy Spinach Soup

Servings: 8    Cooking Time: 3 Hours
**Ingredients:**
- 3 cups frozen spinach, chopped, thawed and drained
- 8 oz cheddar cheese, shredded
- 1 egg, lightly beaten
- 10 oz can cream of chicken soup
- 8 oz cream cheese, softened

**Directions:**
Add spinach to a large bowl. Purée the spinach.    Add egg, chicken soup, cream cheese, and pepper to the spinach purée and mix well.    Transfer spinach mixture to a crock pot.    Cover and cook on low for 3 hours. Stir in cheddar cheese and serve.
**Nutrition Info:**Calories 256 Fat 21.9 g Carbohydrates 4.1 g Sugar 0.5 g Protein 11.1 g Cholesterol 84 mg

## Cream Of Tomato Soup

Servings: 2    Cooking Time: 15 Minutes
**Ingredients:**
- 1lb fresh tomatoes, chopped
- 1.5 cups low sodium tomato puree
- 1tbsp black pepper

**Directions:**
Mix all the ingredients in your Instant Pot.    Cook on Stew for 15 minutes.    Release the pressure naturally. Blend.
**Nutrition Info:**Calories: 20; Carbs: 2; Sugar: 1; Fat: 0; Protein: 3; GL: 1

## Tasty Basil Tomato Soup

Servings: 6    Cooking Time: 6 Hours
**Ingredients:**
- 28 oz can whole peeled tomatoes
- 1/2 cup fresh basil leaves
- 4 cups chicken stock
- 1 tsp red pepper flakes
- 3 garlic cloves, peeled
- 2 onions, diced
- 3 carrots, peeled and diced
- 3 Tbsp olive oil
- 1 tsp salt

**Directions:**
Add all ingredients to a crock pot and stir well.    Cover and cook on low for 6 hours.    Purée the soup until smooth using an immersion blender.    Season soup with pepper and salt.    Serve and enjoy.
**Nutrition Info:**Calories 126 Fat 7.5 g Carbohydrates 13.3 g Sugar 7 g Protein 2.5 g Cholesterol 0 mg

## Fake-on Stew

Servings: 2    Cooking Time: 25 Minutes
**Ingredients:**
- 0.5lb soy bacon
- 1lb chopped vegetables
- 1 cup low sodium vegetable broth
- 1tbsp nutritional yeast

**Directions:**
Mix all the ingredients in your Instant Pot.    Cook on Stew for 25 minutes.    Release the pressure naturally.
**Nutrition Info:** Calories: 200; Carbs: 12; Sugar: 3; Fat: 7; Protein: 41; GL: 5

## Coconut Chicken Soup

Servings: 4    Cooking Time: 18 Minutes
**Ingredients:**
- 4 cloves of garlic, minced
- 1-pound chicken breasts, skin-on
- 4 cups of water
- 2 tablespoons olive oil
- 1 onion, diced
- 1 cup of coconut milk
- (finely ground) black pepper and salt as per taste preference
- 2 tablespoons sesame oil

**Directions:**
Arrange Instant Pot over a dry platform in your kitchen. Open its top lid and switch it on.    Find and press "SAUTE" cooking function; add the oil in it and allow it to heat.    In the pot, add the onions, garlic; cook (while stirring) until turns translucent and softened for around 1-2 minutes.    Stir in the chicken breasts; stir, and cook for 2 more minutes.    Pour in water and coconut milk — season to taste.    Close the lid to create a locked chamber; make sure that safety valve is in locking position.    Find and press "MANUAL" cooking function; timer to 15 minutes with default "HIGH" pressure mode.    Allow the pressure to build to cook the ingredients.    After cooking time is over press "CANCEL" setting. Find and press "NPR" cooking function. This setting is for the natural release of inside pressure and it takes around 10 minutes to slowly release pressure.    Slowly open the lid, Drizzle with sesame oil on top.    Take out the cooked in serving plates or serving bowls and enjoy the keto.
**Nutrition Info:** Calories - 328 Fat: 31g Saturated Fat: 6g Trans Fat: 0g Carbohydrates: 6g Fiber: 4g Sodium: 76mg Protein: 21g

## Herb Tomato Soup

Servings: 8    Cooking Time: 6 Hours
**Ingredients:**
- 55 oz can tomatoes, diced
- 1/2 onion, minced
- 2 cups chicken stock
- 1 cup half and half
- 4 Tbsp butter
- 1 bay leaf
- 1/2 tsp black pepper
- 1/2 tsp garlic powder
- 1 tsp oregano
- 1 tsp dried thyme
- 1 cup carrots, diced
- 1/4 tsp black pepper
- 1/2 tsp salt

**Directions:**
Add all ingredients to a crock pot and stir well.    Cover and cook on low for 6 hours.    Discard bay leaf and purée the soup using an immersion blender until smooth. Serve and enjoy.
**Nutrition Info:** Calories 145 Fat 9.4 g Carbohydrates 13.9 g Sugar 7.9 g Protein 3.2 g Cholesterol 26 mg

## Flavorful Broccoli Soup

Servings: 6    Cooking Time: 4 Hours 15 Minutes
**Ingredients:**
- 20 oz broccoli florets
- 4 oz cream cheese
- 8 oz cheddar cheese, shredded
- 1/2 tsp paprika
- 1/2 tsp ground mustard
- 3 cups chicken stock
- 2 garlic cloves, chopped
- 1 onion, diced
- 1 cup carrots, shredded
- 1/4 tsp baking soda
- 1/4 tsp salt

**Directions:**
Add all ingredients except cream cheese and cheddar cheese to a crock pot and stir well.    Cover and cook on low for 4 hours.    Purée the soup using an immersion blender until smooth.    Stir in the cream cheese and cheddar cheese.    Cover and cook on low for 15 minutes longer.    Season with pepper and salt.    Serve and enjoy.
**Nutrition Info:** Calories 275 Fat 19.9 g Carbohydrates 11.9 g Sugar 4 g Protein 14.4 g Cholesterol 60 mg

## Beef And Cabbage Soup

Servings: 6    Cooking Time: 35 Minutes
**Ingredients:**
- 2 tbsp coconut oil
- 1 onion, diced
- 1 clove garlic, minced
- 1 lb ground beef
- 14 oz can diced tomatoes, undrained
- 4 cups water
- Salt and ground black pepper to taste
- 1 head cabbage, chopped

**Directions:**
Preheat the Instant Pot by selecting SAUTÉ. Add and heat the oil.    Add the onion and garlic and sauté for 2 minutes.    Add the beef and cook, stirring, for 2-3 minutes until lightly brown.    Pour in the water and tomatoes. Season with salt and pepper, stir well.    Press the CANCEL key to stop the SAUTÉ function.    Close and lock the lid. Select MANUAL and cook at HIGH pressure for 12 minutes.    When the timer goes off, use a Quick Release. Carefully open the lid.    Add the cabbage, select SAUTÉ and simmer for 5 minutes. Serve.

**Nutrition Info:**Calories 335 Fat 10 g Carbohydrates 13.6 g Sugar 6 g Protein 4.9 g Cholesterol 33 mg

## Shiitake Soup

Servings: 2      Cooking Time: 35 Minutes
**Ingredients:**
- 1 cup shiitake mushrooms
- 1 cup diced vegetables
- 1 cup low sodium vegetable broth
- 2tbsp 5 spice seasoning

**Directions:**
Mix all the ingredients in your Instant Pot.      Cook on Stew for 35 minutes.      Release the pressure naturally.
**Nutrition Info:**Calories: 70; Carbs: 5; Sugar: 1; Fat: 2; Protein: 2; GL: 1

## Sausage & Turnip Soup

Servings: 4      Cooking Time: 20 Minutes
**Ingredients:**
- 3 turnips, chopped
- 2 celery sticks, chopped
- 2 tbsp butter
- 1 tbsp olive oil
- 1 pork sausage, sliced
- 2 cups vegetable broth
- ½ cup sour cream
- 3 green onions, chopped
- 2 cups water
- Salt and black pepper, to taste

**Directions:**
Sauté the green onions in melted butter over medium heat until soft and golden, about 3-4 minutes. Add celery and turnip, and cook for another 5 minutes. Pour over the vegetable broth and water over.      Bring to a boil, simmer covered, and cook for about 20 minutes until the vegetables are tender. Remove from heat. Puree the soup with a hand blender until smooth. Add sour cream and adjust the seasoning. Warm the olive oil in a skillet. Add the pork sausage and cook for 5 minutes. Serve the soup in deep bowls topped with pork sausage.
**Nutrition Info:**Calories 275, Fat: 23.1g, Net Carbs: 6.4g, Protein: 7.4g

## Simple Chicken Soup

Servings: 4      Cooking Time: 25 Minutes
**Ingredients:**
- 2 frozen, boneless chicken breasts
- 4 medium-sized potatoes, cut into chunks
- 3 carrots, peeled and cut into chunks
- ½ big onion, diced
- 2 cups chicken stock
- 2 cups water
- Salt and ground black pepper to taste

**Directions:**
In the Instant Pot, combine the chicken breasts, potatoes, carrots, onion, stock, water, salt and pepper to taste. Close and lock the lid. Select MANUAL and cook at HIGH pressure for 25 minutes.      Once timer goes off, allow to Naturally Release for 10 minutes, and then

release any remaining pressure manually. Uncover the pot.      Serve.
**Nutrition Info:**Calories 301 Fat 27.2 g Carbohydrates 13.6 g Sugar 6 g Protein 4.9 g Cholesterol 33 mg

## Black Bean Soup

Servings: 4      Cooking Time: 10 Minutes
**Ingredients:**
- 1 tsp. cinnamon powder
- 32 oz. low-sodium chicken stock
- 1 chopped yellow onion
- 1 chopped sweet potato
- 38 oz. no-salt-added, drained and rinsed canned black beans
- 2 tsps. organic olive oil

**Directions:**
Heat up a pot using the oil over medium heat, add onion and cinnamon, stir and cook for 6 minutes.      Add black beans, stock and sweet potato, stir, cook for 14 minutes, puree utilizing an immersion blender, divide into bowls and serve for lunch.      Enjoy!
**Nutrition Info:**Calories: 221, Fat:3 g,Carbs:15 g, Protein:7 g, Sugars:4 g, Sodium:511 mg

## Thick Creamy Broccoli Cheese Soup

Servings: 4      Cooking Time: 10 Minutes
**Ingredients:**
- 1 tbsp olive oil
- 2 tbsp peanut butter
- ¾ cup heavy cream
- 1 onion, diced
- 1 garlic, minced
- 4 cups chopped broccoli
- 4 cups veggie broth
- 2 ¾ cups cheddar cheese, grated
- ¼ cup cheddar cheese to garnish
- Salt and black pepper, to taste
- ½ bunch fresh mint, chopped

**Directions:**
Warm olive oil and peanut butter in a pot over medium heat. Sauté onion and garlic for 3 minutes or until tender, stirring occasionally. Season with salt and black pepper. Add the broth and broccoli and bring to a boil.      Reduce the heat and simmer for 10 minutes. Puree the soup with a hand blender until smooth. Add in the cheese and cook about 1 minute. Stir in the heavy cream. Serve in bowls with the reserved grated cheddar cheese and sprinkled with fresh mint.
**Nutrition Info:**Calories 552, Fat: 49.5g, Net Carbs: 6.9g, Protein: 25g

## Delicious Chicken Soup

Servings: 4      Cooking Time: 4 Hours 30 Minutes
**Ingredients:**
- 1 lb chicken breasts, boneless and skinless
- 2 Tbsp fresh basil, chopped
- 1 1/2 cups mozzarella cheese, shredded
- 2 garlic cloves, minced
- 1 Tbsp Parmesan cheese, grated
- 2 Tbsp dried basil

- 2 cups chicken stock
- 28 oz tomatoes, diced
- 1/4 tsp pepper
- 1/2 tsp salt

**Directions:**
Add chicken, Parmesan cheese, dried basil, tomatoes, garlic, pepper, and salt to a crock pot and stir well to combine.     Cover and cook on low for 4 hours.     Add fresh basil and mozzarella cheese and stir well.     Cover again and cook for 30 more minutes or until cheese is melted.     Remove chicken from the crock pot and shred using forks.     Return shredded chicken to the crock pot and stir to mix.     Serve and enjoy.

**Nutrition Info:**Calories 299 Fat 11.6 g Carbohydrates 9.3 g Sugar 5.6 g Protein 38.8 g Cholesterol 108 mg

## Chicken And Dill Soup

Servings: 6     Cooking Time: 10 Minutes

**Ingredients:**
- 1 c. chopped yellow onion
- 1 whole chicken
- 1 lb. sliced carrots
- 6 c. low-sodium veggie stock
- ¼ tsp. black pepper and salt
- ½ c. chopped red onion
- 2 tsps. chopped dill

**Directions:**
Put chicken in a pot, add water to pay for, give your boil over medium heat, cook first hour, transfer to a cutting board, discard bones, shred the meat, strain the soup, get it back on the pot, heat it over medium heat and add the chicken.     Also add the carrots, yellow onion, red onion, a pinch of salt, black pepper and also the dill, cook for fifteen minutes, ladle into bowls and serve.     Enjoy!

**Nutrition Info:**Calories: 202, Fat:6 g, Carbs:8 g, Protein:12 g, Sugars:6 g, Sodium:514 mg

## Broccoli Stilton Soup

Servings: 2     Cooking Time: 35 Minutes

**Ingredients:**
- 1lb chopped broccoli
- 0.5lb chopped vegetables
- 1 cup low sodium vegetable broth
- 1 cup Stilton

**Directions:**
Mix all the ingredients in your Instant Pot.     Cook on Stew for 35 minutes.     Release the pressure naturally. Blend the soup.

**Nutrition Info:**Calories: 280; Carbs: 9; Sugar: 2; Fat: 22; Protein: 13; GL: 4

## Creamy Broccoli Cauliflower Soup

Servings: 6     Cooking Time: 6 Hours

**Ingredients:**
- 2 cups cauliflower florets, chopped
- 3 cups broccoli florets, chopped
- 3 1/2 cups chicken stock
- 1 large carrot, diced
- 1/2 cup shallots, diced
- 2 garlic cloves, minced

- 1 cup plain yogurt
- 6 oz cheddar cheese, shredded
- 1 cup coconut milk
- Pepper
- Salt

**Directions:**
Add all ingredients except milk, cheese, and yogurt to a crock pot and stir well.     Cover and cook on low for 6 hours.     Purée the soup using an immersion blender until smooth.     Add cheese, milk, and yogurt and blend until smooth and creamy.     Season with pepper and salt.     Serve and enjoy.

**Nutrition Info:**Calories 281 Fat 20 g Carbohydrates 14.4 g Sugar 6.9 g Protein 13.1 g Cholesterol 32 mg

## Zoodle Won-ton Soup

Servings: 2     Cooking Time: 5 Minutes

**Ingredients:**
- 1lb spiralized zucchini
- 1 pack unfried won-tons
- 1 cup low sodium beef broth
- 2tbsp soy sauce

**Directions:**
Mix all the ingredients in your Instant Pot.     Cook on Stew for 5 minutes.     Release the pressure naturally.

**Nutrition Info:**Calories: 300; Carbs: 6; Sugar: 1; Fat: 9; Protein: 43; GL: 2

## Pumpkin Spice Soup

Servings: 2     Cooking Time: 35 Minutes

**Ingredients:**
- 1lb cubed pumpkin
- 1 cup low sodium vegetable broth
- 2tbsp mixed spice

**Directions:**
Mix all the ingredients in your Instant Pot.     Cook on Stew for 35 minutes.     Release the pressure naturally. Blend the soup.

**Nutrition Info:**Calories: 100; Carbs: 7; Sugar: 1; Fat: 2; Protein: 3; GL: 1

## Kidney Bean Stew

Servings: 2     Cooking Time: 15 Minutes

**Ingredients:**
- 1lb cooked kidney beans
- 1 cup tomato passata
- 1 cup low sodium beef broth
- 3tbsp Italian herbs

**Directions:**
Mix all the ingredients in your Instant Pot.     Cook on Stew for 15 minutes.     Release the pressure naturally.

**Nutrition Info:**Calories: 270; Carbs: 16; Sugar: 3; Fat: 10; Protein: 23; GL: 8

## Cream Zucchini Soup

Servings: 4     Cooking Time: 8 Minutes

**Ingredients:**
- 2 cups vegetable stock
- 2 garlic cloves, crushed
- 1 tablespoon butter

- 4 (preferably medium size) zucchinis, peeled and chopped
- 1 small onion, chopped
- 2 cups heavy cream
- 1/2 teaspoon dried oregano, (finely ground)
- 1/2 teaspoon black pepper, (finely ground)
- 1 teaspoon dried parsley, (finely ground)
- 1 teaspoon of sea salt
- Lemon juice (optional)

**Directions:**
Arrange Instant Pot over a dry platform in your kitchen. Open its top lid and switch it on. Find and press "SAUTE" cooking function; add the butter in it and allow it to melt. In the pot, add the onions, zucchini, garlic; cook (while stirring) until turns translucent and softened for around 2-3 minutes. Add the vegetable broth and sprinkle with salt, oregano, pepper, and parsley; gently stir to mix well. Close the lid to create a locked chamber; make sure that safety valve is in locking position. Find and press "MANUAL" cooking function; timer to 5 minutes with default "HIGH" pressure mode. Allow the pressure to build to cook the ingredients. After cooking time is over press "CANCEL" setting. Find and press "QPR" cooking function. This setting is for quick release of inside pressure. Slowly open the lid, take out the cooked in serving plates or serving bowls, and enjoy the keto . Top with some lemon juice.

**Nutrition Info:**Calories - 264 Fat: 26g Saturated Fat: 7g Trans Fat: 0g Carbohydrates: 11g Fiber: 3g Sodium: 564mg Protein: 4g

## Spinach & Basil Chicken Soup

Servings: 4      Cooking Time: 10 Minutes
**Ingredients:**
- 1 cup spinach
- 2 cups cooked and shredded chicken
- 4 cups chicken broth
- 1 cup cheddar cheese, shredded

- 4 ounces' cream cheese
- ½ tsp chili powder
- ½ tsp ground cumin
- ½ tsp fresh parsley, chopped
- Salt and black pepper, to taste

**Directions:**
In a pot, add the chicken broth and spinach, bring to a boil and cook for 5-8 minutes. Transfer to a food processor, add in the cream cheese and pulse until smooth. Return the mixture to a pot and place over medium heat. Cook until hot, but do not bring to a boil. Add chicken, chili powder, and cumin and cook for about 3-5 minutes, or until it is heated through. Stir in cheddar cheese and season with salt and pepper. Serve hot in bowls sprinkled with parsley.

**Nutrition Info:**Calories 351, Fat: 22.4g, Net Carbs: 4.3g, Protein: 21.6g

## Easy Wonton Soup

Servings: 6      Cooking Time: 20 Minutes
**Ingredients:**
- 4 sliced scallions
- ¼ tsp. ground white pepper
- 2 c. sliced fresh mushrooms
- 4 minced garlic cloves
- 6 oz. dry whole-grain yolk-free egg noodles
- ½ lb. lean ground pork
- 1 tbsp. minced fresh ginger
- 8 c. low-sodium chicken broth

**Directions:**
Place a stockpot over medium heat. Add the ground pork, ginger, and garlic and sauté for 5 minutes. Drain any excess fat, then return to stovetop. Add the broth and bring to a boil. Once boiling, stir in the mushrooms, noodles, and white pepper. Cover and simmer for 10 minutes. Remove pot from heat. Stir in the scallions and serve immediately.

**Nutrition Info:**Calories: 143, Fat:4 g, Carbs:14 g, Protein:12 g, Sugars:0.8 g, Sodium:901 mg

# Snack And Desserts Recipes

## Lemon Fat Bombs

Servings: 10     Cooking Time: 0 Minutes
**Ingredients:**
- Coconut butter, full-fat: 3/4 cup
- Avocado oil: 1/4 cup
- Lemon juice: 3 tablespoons
- Zest of lemon: 1
- Coconut cream, full-fat: 1 tablespoon
- Erythritol sweetener: 1 tablespoon
- Vanilla extract, unsweetened: 1 teaspoon
- Salt: 1/8 teaspoon

**Directions:**
Place all the ingredients for fat bombs in a blender and pulse until well combined.     Take a baking dish, line it with parchment sheet, then transfer the fat bomb mixture on the sheet and place the sheet into the freezer for 45 minutes until firm enough to shape into balls. Then remove the baking sheet from the freezer, roll the fat bomb mixture into ten balls, and arrange the fat bombs on the baking sheet in a single layer.     Return the baking sheet into the freezer, let chilled until hard and set, and then store in the freezer for up to 2 months. Serve when required.
**Nutrition Info:**Calories: 164 Fat: 16.7 g Protein: 1.3 g Net Carbs: 0.4 g Fiber: 3 g

## Garden Patch Sandwiches On Multigrain Bread

Servings: 4     Cooking Time: 0 Minutes
**Ingredients:**
- 1pound extra-firm tofu, drained and patted dry
- 1 medium red bell pepper, finely chopped
- 1 celery rib, finely chopped
- 3 green onions, minced
- ¼ cup shelled sunflower seeds
- ½ cup vegan mayonnaise, homemade or store-bought
- ½ teaspoon salt
- ½ teaspoon celery salt
- ¼ teaspoon freshly ground black pepper
- 8 slices whole grain bread
- 4 (¼-inch) slices ripe tomato
- 4 lettuce leaves

**Directions:**
Preparing the Ingredients     Smash the tofu and place it in a large bowl. Add the bell pepper, celery, green onions, and sunflower seeds. Stir in the mayonnaise, salt, celery salt, and pepper and mix until well combined.     Finish and Serve     Toast the bread, if desired. Spread the mixture evenly onto 4 slices of the bread.
**Nutrition Info:**166 Cal 15 g Fats 6.5 g Protein 2 g Net Carb 0 g Fiber

## Sesame Almond Fat Bombs

Servings: 16     Cooking Time: 0 Minutes
**Ingredients:**

- 1 cup coconut oil
- 1 cup smooth almond butter
- ½ cup unsweetened cocoa powder
- ¼ cup almond flour
- Liquid stevia extract, to taste
- ½ cup toasted sesame seeds

**Directions:**
Combine the coconut oil and almond butter in a small saucepan.     Cook over low heat until melted, then whisk in the cocoa powder, almond flour, and liquid stevia.     Remove from heat and let cool until it hardens slightly.     Divide the mixture into 16 even pieces and roll into balls.     Roll the balls in the toasted sesame seeds and chill until ready to eat.
**Nutrition Info:**260 calories 26g fat 4g protein 6g carbs 2g fiber 4g net carbs

## Sugar Free Carrot Cake

Servings: 8     Cooking Time: 4 Hours
**Ingredients:**
- For Carrot cake:
- 2 eggs
- 1 1/2 almond flour
- 1/2 cup butter, melted
- ¼ cup heavy cream
- 1 teaspoon baking powder
- 1 teaspoon vanilla extract or almond extract, optional
- 1 cup sugar substitute
- 1 cup carrots, finely shredded
- 1 teaspoon cinnamon
- ¼ teaspoon nutmeg
- 1/8 teaspoon allspice
- 1 teaspoon ginger
- 1/2 teaspoon baking soda
- For cream cheese frosting:
- 1 cup confectioner's sugar substitute
- ¼ cup butter, softened
- 1 teaspoon almond extract
- 4 oz. cream cheese, softened

**Directions:**
Grease a loaf pan well and then set it aside.     Using a mixer, combine butter together with eggs, vanilla, sugar substitute and heavy cream in a mixing bowl, until well blended.     Combine almond flour together with baking powder, spices and the baking soda in a another bowl until well blended.     When done, combine the wet ingredients together with the dry ingredients until well blended, and then stir in carrots.     Pour the mixer into the prepared loaf pan, and then place the pan into a slow cooker on a trivet. Add 1 cup water inside.     Cook for about 4-5 hours on low. Be aware that the cake will be very moist.     When the cooking time is over, let the cake cool completely.     To prepare the cream cheese frosting: blend the cream cheese together with extract, butter and powdered sugar substitute until frosting is formed. Top the cake with the frosting.

**Nutrition Info:** 299 calories; 25.4 g fat; 15 g total carbs; 4 g protein

## Spice Cake

Servings: 10    Cooking Time: 50 Minutes
**Ingredients:**
- Almond flour: 2 cups
- Erythritol sweetener: ½ cup
- Baking powder: 2 teaspoons
- Ground cinnamon: 1 teaspoon
- Ground ginger: 1 teaspoon
- Ground cloves: ¼ teaspoon
- Salt: ¼ teaspoon
- Eggs: 2
- Butter, unsalted, melted: 1/3 cup
- Water, divided: 1 1/3 cup
- Vanilla extract, unsweetened: ½ teaspoon
- Chopped toasted pecans: 3 tablespoons

**Directions:**
Place all the ingredients in a bowl, reserving 1 cup water and pecans, and stir well using a hand mixer until incorporated and a smooth batter comes together. Take a 7-inch baking pan, spoon the batter on it, then smooth the top, sprinkle with pecans and cover the pan with aluminum foil.    Switch on the instant pot, pour in water, insert a trivet stand and place pan on it.    Shut the instant pot with its lid in the sealed position, then press the 'cake' button, press '+/-' to set the cooking time to 40 minutes and cook at high-pressure setting; when the pressure builds in the pot, the cooking timer will start. When the instant pot buzzes, press the 'keep warm' button, release pressure naturally for 10 minutes, then do a quick pressure release and open the lid.    Take out the pan, uncover it, invert the pan on a plate to take out the cake and let cool for 10 minutes.    Spread cream on top of the cake, then cut into slices and serve.
**Nutrition Info:** Calories: 229 Fat: 21 g Protein: 6 g Net Carbs: 2 g Fiber: 0 g

## Creamy Chocolate Pie Ice Pops

Servings: 9    Cooking Time: 15 Minutes
**Ingredients:**
- 1 (4-serving size) package fat-free, sugar-free, reduced-calorie chocolate instant pudding mix
- 2 cups unsweetened almond milk or fat-free milk
- 1 cup frozen light whipped topping, thawed
- 1 oz. dark chocolate, melted
- 1 tbsp. crushed graham crackers

**Directions:**
Whisk together almond milk and pudding mix for 2 to 3 minutes in a medium bowl or until thick. Fold in whipped topping.    Ladle mixture into nine 3-oz. paper cups or ice pop molds. Insert sticks into the molds. In case you're using paper cups, use foil to cover each cup, make a small slit in the foil and then insert a wooden stick into each pop. Freeze overnight or until firm.    Unmold the pops. As you work with one pop at a time, drizzle with the melted chocolate and immediately sprinkle with graham crackers.
**Nutrition Info:** Calories: 60 calories; Total Carbohydrate: 9 g Cholesterol: 0 mg Total Fat: 3 g

Fiber: 1 g Protein: 1 g Sodium: 175 mg Sugar: 2 g Saturated Fat: 2 g

## Caramel Popcorn

Servings: 20    Cooking Time: 10 Minutes
**Ingredients:**
- 1 cup butter
- 2 cups brown sugar
- 1/2 cup corn syrup
- 1 tsp. salt
- 1/2 tsp. baking soda
- 1 tsp. vanilla extract
- 5 quarts popped popcorn

**Directions:**
Start preheating the oven to 250°F (95°C). In a very big bowl, put popcorn.    Melt butter over medium heat in a medium-sized saucepan. Mix in salt, corn syrup, and brown sugar. Boil it, tossing continually. Boil without tossing for 4 minutes. Take away from the heat and mix in vanilla and soda. Add to the popcorn in a thin flow, tossing to blend.    Put in 2 big shallow cookie sheets and bake in the preheated oven for 1 hour, tossing every 15 minutes. Take out of the oven and let cool fully and then crumble into chunks.
**Nutrition Info:** Calories: 253 calories Total Carbohydrate: 32.8 g Cholesterol: 24 mg Total Fat: 14 g Protein: 0.9 g Sodium: 340 mg

## Tiramisu Shots

Servings: 4    Cooking Time: 10 Minutes
**Ingredients:**
- 1 pack silken tofu
- 1 oz. dark chocolate, finely chopped
- ¼ cup sugar substitute
- 1 teaspoon lemon juice
- ¼ cup brewed espresso
- Pinch salt
- 24 slices angel food cake
- Cocoa powder (unsweetened)

**Directions:**
Add tofu, chocolate, sugar substitute, lemon juice, espresso and salt in a food processor.    Pulse until smooth.    Add angel food cake pieces into shot glasses. Drizzle with the cocoa powder.    Pour the tofu mixture on top.    Top with the remaining angel food cake pieces. Chill for 30 minutes and serve.
**Nutrition Info:** Calories 75 Total Fat 1.8 g Total Carbohydrate 12 g Protein 2.9 g

## Fruit Kebab

Servings: 12    Cooking Time: 0 Minutes
**Ingredients:**
- 3 apples
- ¼ cup orange juice
- 1 ½ lb. watermelon
- ¾ cup blueberries

**Directions:**
Use a star-shaped cookie cutter to cut out stars from the apple and watermelon.    Soak the apple stars in orange juice.    Thread the apple stars, watermelon stars and

blueberries into skewers.    Refrigerate for 30 minutes before serving.
**Nutrition Info:**Calories 52 Total Fat 0 g Saturated Fat 0 g Cholesterol 0 mg Sodium 1 mg Total Carbohydrate 14 g Dietary Fiber 2 g Total Sugars 10 g Protein 1 g Potassium 134 mg

## Cheese Berry Fat Bomb

Servings: 12    Cooking Time: 5 Minutes
**Ingredients:**
- 1 cup fresh berries, wash
- 1/2 cup coconut oil
- 1 1/2 cup cream cheese, softened
- 1 tbsp vanilla
- 2 tbsp swerve

**Directions:**
Add all ingredients to the blender and blend until smooth and combined.    Spoon mixture into small candy molds and refrigerate until set.    Serve and enjoy.
**Nutrition Info:**Calories 175 Fat 17 g Carbohydrates 2 g Sugar 1 g Protein 2.1 g Cholesterol 29 mg

## Tamari Toasted Almonds

Servings: ½    Cooking Time: 8 Minutes
**Ingredients:**
- ½ cup raw almonds, or sunflower seeds
- 2 tablespoons tamari, or soy sauce
- 1 teaspoon toasted sesame oil

**Directions:**
Preparing the Ingredients    Heat a dry skillet to medium-high heat, then add the almonds, stirring frequently to keep them from burning. Once the almonds are toasted—7-8 minutes for almonds, or 34 minutes for sunflower seeds—pour the tamari and sesame oil into the hot skillet and stir to coat.    You can turn off the heat, and as the almonds cool the tamari mixture will stick and dry on to the nuts.
**Nutrition Info:**Calories: 89 Total fat: 8g Carbs: 3g Fiber: 2g Protein: 4g

## Choco Peppermint Cake

Servings: 4    Cooking Time: 10 Minutes
**Ingredients:**
- Cooking spray
- ⅓ cup oil
- 15 oz. package chocolate cake mix
- 3 eggs, beaten
- 1 cup water
- ¼ teaspoon peppermint extract

**Directions:**
Spray slow cooker with oil.    Mix all the ingredients in a bowl.    Use an electric mixer on medium speed setting to mix ingredients for 2 minutes.    Pour mixture into the slow cooker.    Cover the pot and cook on low for 3 hours.    Let cool before slicing and serving.
**Nutrition Info:**Calories 185 Total Fat 7.4 g Total Carbohydrate 27 g Protein 3.8 g

## Frozen Lemon & Blueberry

Servings: 4    Cooking Time: 10 Minutes

**Ingredients:**
- 6 cup fresh blueberries
- 8 sprigs fresh thyme
- ¾ cup light brown sugar
- 1 teaspoon lemon zest
- ¼ cup lemon juice
- 2 cups water

**Directions:**
Add blueberries, thyme and sugar in a pan over medium heat.    Cook for 6 to 8 minutes.    Transfer mixture to a blender.    Remove thyme sprigs.    Stir in the remaining ingredients.    Pulse until smooth.    Strain mixture and freeze for 1 hour.
**Nutrition Info:**Calories 78 Total Fat 0 g Total Carbohydrate 20 g Protein 3 g

## Pumpkin & Banana Ice Cream

Servings: 4    Cooking Time: 10 Minutes
**Ingredients:**
- 15 oz. pumpkin puree
- 4 bananas, sliced and frozen
- 1 teaspoon pumpkin pie spice
- Chopped pecans

**Directions:**
Add pumpkin puree, bananas and pumpkin pie spice in a food processor.    Pulse until smooth.    Chill in the refrigerator.    Garnish with pecans.
**Nutrition Info:**Calories 71 Total Fat 0.4 g Total Carbohydrate 18 g Protein 1.2 g

## Coconut Chia Pudding

Servings: 6    Cooking Time: 0 Minutes
**Ingredients:**
- 2 ¼ cup canned coconut milk
- 1 teaspoon vanilla extract
- Pinch salt
- ½ cup chia seeds

**Directions:**
Combine the coconut milk, vanilla, and salt in a bowl. Stir well and sweeten with stevia to taste.    Whisk in the chia seeds and chill overnight.    Spoon into bowls and serve with chopped nuts or fruit.
**Nutrition Info:**300 calories 27.5g fat 6g protein 14.5g carbs 10g fiber 4.5g net carbs

## Strawberries In Honey Yogurt Dip

Servings: 4    Cooking Time: 0 Minutes
**Ingredients:**
- 1 cup plain yogurt, low-fat
- 1 tablespoon of orange juice
- 1 to 2 teaspoons of honey
- Ground cinnamon
- 1 quart of fresh strawberries (remove stems)

**Directions:**
Combine first four ingredients to make a sauce. Pour over strawberries and serve.
**Nutrition Info:**Calories: 88 Carbohydrates: 16 g Fiber: 4 g Fats: 1 g Sodium: 41 mg Protein: 4 g Diabetic Exchange: 1/2 Milk, 1 Fruit

## Mortadella & Bacon Balls

Servings: 2    Cooking Time: 20 Minutes

**Ingredients:**

- 4 ounces Mortadella sausage
- 4 bacon slices, cooked and crumbled
- 2 tbsp almonds, chopped
- ½ tsp Dijon mustard
- 3 ounces' cream cheese

**Directions:**

Combine the mortadella and almonds in the bowl of your food processor. Pulse until smooth. Whisk the cream cheese and mustard in another bowl. Make balls out of the mortadella mixture.    Make a thin cream cheese layer over. Coat with bacon, arrange on a plate and chill before serving.

**Nutrition Info:**Calories 547 Fat: 51g Net Carbs: 3.4g Protein: 21.5g

## Lemon Cake

Servings: 9    Cooking Time: 20 Minutes

**Ingredients:**

- 2 Medium lemons
- 4 Large eggs
- 2 Tablespoons of almond butter
- 2 Tablespoons of avocado oil
- 1/3 cup of coconut flour
- 4-5 tablespoons of honey (or another sweetener of your choice)
- 1/2 tablespoon of baking soda

**Directions:**

Preheat your oven to a temperature of about 350 F. Crack the eggs in a large bowl and set two egg whites aside.    Whisk the 2 whites of eggs with the egg yolks, the honey, the oil, the almond butter, the lemon zest and the juice and whisk very well together.    Combine the baking soda with the coconut flour and gradually add this dry mixture to the wet ingredients and keep whisking for a couple of minutes.    Beat the two eggs with a hand mixer and beat the egg into foam.    Add the white egg foam gradually to the mixture with a silicone spatula.    Transfer your obtained batter to tray covered with a baking paper.    Bake your cake for about 20 to 22 minutes.    Let the cake cool for 5 minutes; then slice your cake.    Serve and enjoy your delicious cake!

**Nutrition Info:**Calories: 164| Fat: 12g | Carbohydrates: 7.1 | Fiber: 2.7g |Protein: 10.9g

## Green Fruity Smoothie

Servings: 2    Cooking Time: 10 Minutes

**Ingredients:**

- 1 cup frozen mango, peeled, pitted, and chopped
- 1 large frozen banana, peeled
- 2 cups fresh baby spinach
- 1 scoop unsweetened vegan vanilla protein powder
- ¼ cup pumpkin seeds
- 2 tablespoons hemp hearts
- 1½ cups unsweetened almond milk

**Directions:**

In a high-speed blender, place all the ingredients and pulse until creamy.    Pour into two glasses and serve immediately.

**Nutrition Info:**Calories 355 Total Fat 16.1 g Saturated Fat 2.4 g Cholesterol 0 mg Sodium 295 mg Total Carbs 34.6 g Fiber 6.2 g Sugar 19.9 g Protein 23.4 g

## Baked Creamy Custard With Maple

Servings: 6    Cooking Time: 15 Minutes

**Ingredients:**

- 2 1/2 cups half-and-half, fat-free
- 1/2 cup egg substitute, cholesterol-free
- 1/4 cup sugar
- 2 teaspoons vanilla
- Dash ground nutmeg
- 3 cups of boiling water
- 2 tablespoons of maple syrup

**Directions:**

Spray 6 ramekins or custard cups with light non-stick cooking spray. Preheat your oven to 325ºF.    Combine first five ingredients and mix well. Pour into your ramekins.    Pour the boiling water in a 13x9-inch baking dish. Place the ramekins in the dish and bake 1 hour 15 minutes.    Cool the ramekins on a cooling rack. Cover with a plastic wrap and chill in the fridge overnight. Drizzle with maple syrup before serving.

**Nutrition Info:**Calories: 131 Carbohydrates: 23 g Fiber: 0 g Fats: 1 g Sodium: 139 mg Protein: 5 g

## Lemon Cookies

Servings: 6    Cooking Time: 12 Minutes

**Ingredients:**

- ¼ cup unsweetened applesauce
- 1 cup cashew butter
- 1 teaspoon fresh lemon zest, grated finely
- 2 tablespoons fresh lemon juice
- Pinch of sea salt

**Directions:**

Preheat the oven to 350 degrees F. Line a large cookie sheet with parchment paper.    In a food processor, add all ingredients and pulse until smooth.    With a tablespoon, place the mixture onto prepared cookie sheet in a single layer.    Bake for about 12 minutes or until golden brown.    Remove from oven and place the cookie sheet onto a wire rack to cool for about 5 minutes.    Carefully invert the cookies onto wire rack to cool completely before serving.    Meal Prep Tip: Store these cookies in an airtight container, by placing parchment papers between the cookies to avoid the sticking. These cookies can be stored in the refrigerator for up to 2 weeks.

**Nutrition Info:**Calories 257 Total Fat 21.9 g Saturated Fat 4.2 g Cholesterol 0 mg Total Carbs 13.1 g Sugar 1.2 g Fiber 1 g Sodium 47 mg Potassium 248 mg Protein 7.6 g

## Pineapple Nice Cream

Servings: 6    Cooking Time: 15 Minutes

**Ingredients:**

- 1 16-oz. package frozen pineapple chunks
- 1 cup frozen mango chunks or 1 large mango, peeled, seeded and chopped

- 1 tbsp. lemon juice or lime juice

**Directions:**

In a food processor, process the mango, lemon or lime juice, and pineapple until creamy and smooth. You can add a 1/4 cup of water if the mango is frozen. Serve it immediately if you want to have the best texture.

**Nutrition Info:**Calories: 55 calories; Total Carbohydrate: 14 g Cholesterol: 0 mg Total Fat: 0 g Fiber: 2 g Protein: 1 g Sodium: 1 mg Sugar: 11 g Saturated Fat: 0 g

## Garden Salad Wraps

Servings: 4      Cooking Time: 10 Minutes

**Ingredients:**

- 6 tablespoons extra-virgin olive oil
- 1-pound extra-firm tofu, drained, patted dry, and cut into ½-inch strips
- 1 tablespoon soy sauce
- ¼ cup apple cider vinegar
- 1 teaspoon yellow or spicy brown mustard
- ½ teaspoon salt
- ¼ teaspoon freshly ground black pepper
- 3 cups shredded romaine lettuce
- 3 ripe Roma tomatoes, finely chopped
- 1 large carrot, shredded
- 1 medium English cucumber, peeled and chopped
- ⅓ cup minced red onion
- ¼ cup sliced pitted green olives
- 4 (10-inch) whole-grain flour tortillas or lavish flatbread

**Directions:**

Preparing the Ingredients     Cook the tofu until golden brown in a large skillet with Over medium heat. Sprinkle with soy sauce and set aside to cool.     In a small bowl, combine the vinegar, mustard, salt and pepper with the remaining 4 tablespoons oil, stirring to blend well. Set aside.     Finish and Serve     combine the cucumber, onion, lettuce, tomatoes, carrot, and olives in a large bowl. Pour on the dressing.     Put 1 tortilla on a work surface and spread with about one-quarter of the salad. Place a few strips of tofu on the tortilla and roll up tightly. Slice in half.

**Nutrition Info:**191 Cal 16.6 g Fats 9.6 g Protein 0.8 g Net Carb 0.2 g Fiber

## Roasted Eggplant Spread

Servings: 2      Cooking Time: 20 Minutes

**Ingredients:**

- 1 eggplant, medium, cut into small 1 inch pieces
- 2 red peppers, cut into 1-inch pieces
- 1 red onion, cut into 1-inch pieces
- 1 tablespoon tomato
- 4 toasted baguette slices
- What you will need from the store cupboard:
- 3 garlic cloves, minced
- 3 tablespoons of olive oil
- ½ teaspoon pepper
- ½ teaspoon salt
- Cooking spray

**Directions:**

Preheat your oven to 350 ºF.     Mix the olive oil, cloves, salt, and pepper.     Keep vegetables in your bowl. Now toss with the oil mix.     Transfer to your baking pan where you have applied cooking spray     Roast the vegetables till they get soft and are slightly brown. Now keep in a food processor.     Add the tomato and pulse until it blends. The mixture must be chunky. Transfer to your bowl. Serve with the baguette.

**Nutrition Info:**Calories 84 Carbohydrates 9g Fiber 3g Sugar 0.5g Cholesterol 0mg Total Fat 5g Protein 1g

## Chocolate Muffins

Servings: 8      Cooking Time: 30 Minutes

**Ingredients:**

- Pumpkin, chopped, steamed: 2 cups
- Coconut flour: 1/2 cup
- Salt: 1/8 teaspoon
- Erythritol sweetener: 4 tablespoons
- Cacao powder, unsweetened: 1 cup
- Collagen protein powder: 1/2 cup
- Baking soda: 1 teaspoon
- Cacao butter, melted: 4.6 ounces
- Avocado oil: 1/2 cup
- Apple cider vinegar: 2 teaspoons
- Vanilla extract, unsweetened: 3 teaspoons
- Eggs, pastured: 3

**Directions:**

Set oven to 350 degrees F and let preheat until muffins are ready to bake.     Add all the ingredients in a food processor or blender, except for collagen, and pulse for 1 to 2 minutes or until well combined and incorporated. Then add collagen and pulse at low speed until just mixed.     Take an eight cups silicon muffin tray, grease the cups with avocado oil and then evenly scoop the batter in them.     Place the muffin tray into the oven and bake the muffins for 30 minutes or until thoroughly cooked and a knife inserted into each muffin comes out clean.     When done, let muffins cool in the pan for 10 minutes, then take them out from the tray and cool on the wire rack.     Place muffins in a large freezer bag or wrap each muffin with a foil and store them in the refrigerator for four days or in the freezer for up to 3 months.     When ready to serve, microwave muffins for 45 seconds to 1 minute or until thoroughly heated and then serve with coconut cream.

**Nutrition Info:**Calories: 111 Fat: 9.9 g Protein: 2.8 g Net Carbs: 3 g Fiber: 1 g

## Dark Chocolate Cake

Servings: 10      Cooking Time: 3 Hours

**Ingredients:**

- 1 cup almond flour
- 3 eggs
- 2 tablespoons almond flour
- 1/4 teaspoon salt
- 1/2 cup Swerve Granular
- 3/4 teaspoon vanilla extract
- 2/3 cup  almond milk, unsweetened
- 1/2 cup cocoa powder
- 6 tablespoons butter, melted
- 1 1/2 teaspoon baking powder

- 3 tablespoon unflavored whey protein powder or egg white protein powder
- 1/3 cup sugar-free chocolate chips, optional

**Directions:**
Grease the slow cooker well. Whisk the almond flour together with cocoa powder, sweetener, whey protein powder, salt and baking powder in a bowl. Then stir in butter along with almond milk, eggs and the vanilla extract until well combined, and then stir in the chocolate chips if desired. When done, pour into the slow cooker. Allow to cook for 2-2 1/2 hours on low. When through, turn off the slow cooker and let the cake cool for about 20-30 minutes. When cooled, cut the cake into pieces and serve warm with lightly sweetened whipped cream. Enjoy!

**Nutrition Info:**205 calories; 17 g fat; 8.4 g total carbs; 12 g protein

## Strawberry & Watermelon Pops

Servings: 6     Cooking Time: 0 Minutes

**Ingredients:**
- ¾ cup strawberries, sliced
- 2 cups watermelon, cubed
- ¼ cup lime juice
- 2 tablespoons brown sugar
- ⅛ teaspoon salt

**Directions:**
Put the strawberries inside popsicle molds. In a blender, pulse the rest of the ingredients until well mixed. Pour the puree into a sieve before pouring into the molds. Freeze for 6 hours.

**Nutrition Info:**Calories 57 Total Fat 0 g Saturated Fat 0 g Cholesterol 0 mg Sodium 180 mg Total Carbohydrate 14 g Dietary Fiber 2 g Total Sugars 11 g Protein 1 g Potassium 180 mg

## Raspberry Almond Tart

Servings: 4     Cooking Time: 23 Minutes

**Ingredients:**
- 5 egg whites
- 1 tsp vanilla
- 1 1/2 cups raspberries
- 1 lemon zest, grated
- 1 cup almond flour
- 1/2 cup Swerve
- 1/2 cup butter, melted
- 1 tsp baking powder

**Directions:**
Preheat the oven to 375 F/ 190 C. Grease tart tin with cooking spray and set aside. In a large bowl, whisk egg whites until foamy. Add sweetener, baking powder, vanilla, lemon zest, and almond flour and mix until well combined. Add melted butter and stir well. Pour batter in tart tin and top with raspberries. Bake in preheated oven for 20-23 minutes. Serve and enjoy.

**Nutrition Info:**Calories 378 Fat 8 g Carbohydrates 14 g Sugar 4 g Protein 11 g Cholesterol 0 mg

## Oatmeal Butterscotch Cookies

Servings: 4 Dozen     Cooking Time: 15 Minutes

**Ingredients:**
- ½ teaspoon cinnamon, ground
- 3 cups oats
- 2 eggs
- What you will need from the store cupboard:
- 1 teaspoon of baking soda
- 1-1/4 all-purpose flour
- 1 cup margarine or butter
- 1 teaspoon vanilla extract
- ½ teaspoon salt

**Directions:**
Preheat your oven to 350 °F. Bring together the baking soda, flour, salt and cinnamon in a bowl. Beat the eggs, vanilla extract and butter in a mixer bowl. Beat in the flour mix gradually. Stir in the oats. Place rounded tablespoons on baking sheets. Bake for 5-6 minutes. Let it cool for a couple of minutes.

**Nutrition Info:**Calories 130 Carbohydrates 16g Cholesterol 20mg Fat 7g Protein 1g Sodium 90mg

## Avocado Mousse

Servings: 3

**Ingredients:**
- 2 ripe Haas avocados, peeled, pitted and chopped roughly
- 1 teaspoon liquid stevia
- 1 teaspoon organic vanilla extract
- Pinch of salt

**Directions:**
In a high-speed blender, add all the ingredients and pulse until smooth. Transfer the pudding into a serving bowl. Cover the bowl and refrigerate to chill for at least 2 hours before serving. Meal Prep Tip: Transfer the mousse into an airtight container. Cover the containers and refrigerate for about 1 day.

**Nutrition Info:**Calories 277 Total Fat 26.1 g Saturated Fat 5.5 g Cholesterol 0 mg Total Carbs 11.7 g Sugar 0.9 g Fiber 8 g Sodium 59 mg Potassium 652 mg Protein 2.6g

## Flourless Chocolate Cake

Servings: 6     Cooking Time: 45 Minutes

**Ingredients:**
- 1/2 Cup of stevia
- 12 Ounces of unsweetened baking chocolate
- 2/3 Cup of ghee
- 1/3 Cup of warm water
- ¼ Teaspoon of salt
- 4 Large pastured eggs
- 2 Cups of boiling water

**Directions:**
Line the bottom of a 9-inch pan of a spring form with a parchment paper. Heat the water in a small pot; then add the salt and the stevia over the water until wait until the mixture becomes completely dissolved. Melt the baking chocolate into a double boiler or simply microwave it for about 30 seconds. Mix the melted chocolate and the butter in a large bowl with an electric mixer. Beat in your hot mixture; then crack in the egg and whisk after adding each of the eggs. Pour the obtained mixture into your prepared spring form tray. Wrap the spring form tray with a foil paper. Place the

spring form tray in a large cake tray and add boiling water right to the outside; make sure the depth doesn't exceed 1 inch. Bake the cake into the water bath for about 45 minutes at a temperature of about 350 F. Remove the tray from the boiling water and transfer to a wire to cool. Let the cake chill for an overnight in the refrigerator. Serve and enjoy your delicious cake!
**Nutrition Info:**Calories: 295| Fat: 26g | Carbohydrates: 6g | Fiber: 4g |Protein: 8g

## Berry Almond Parfait

Servings: 4     Cooking Time: 30 Minutes
**Ingredients:**
- 1-8 ounces' container plain yogurt, low-fat and drained
- 1 cup of sliced strawberries
- 1/2 cup raspberries
- 1/2 cup blueberries
- 1/8 teaspoon of almond extract
- 1 tablespoon pourable sugar substitute + 2 teaspoons, divided
- 2 tablespoons toasted slivered almonds for toppings

**Directions:**
Drain and thicken yogurt in the fridge using a paper towel lined strainer for 2 hours to 24 hours. (Do this the night before). Combine all ingredients but using only 2-teaspoon sugar substitute. Toss lightly to mix. Chill for 30 minutes to 2 hours. Transfer the drained yogurt to a bowl and stir in the remaining sugar substitute. Layer 1/3 cup of berries mixture and half yogurt alternately in 2 parfait glasses. Top with almonds to serve.
**Nutrition Info:**Calories: 220 Carbohydrates: 30 g Fiber: 6 g Fats: 6 g Sodium: 84 mg Protein: 9 g

## Homemade Ice Cream Cake

Servings: 4     Cooking Time: 15 Minutes
**Ingredients:**
- 5 sugar cones, crushed
- 3 tablespoons melted unsalted butter
- 4 cups light ice cream, no-sugar-added and softened, divided
- 1-8 ounces' container whipped topping, reduced-fat and frozen thawed

**Directions:**
Grease a deep pie pan dish with cooking spray. Crush sugar cones in a sealed bag using a rolling pin. Place in a bowl. Stir in the butter until evenly moistened. Use the mixture as your crust. Press onto the bottom of the pan and refrigerate for 20 minutes. Layer 2 cups of the light ice cream over the crust and freeze for 30 minutes or until firm. Spread the remaining light ice cream on top of the frozen first layer and freeze again for another 30 minutes. Spread the whip topping on top then freeze for 2 hours or until it is firm. Let ice cream cake soften for 15 to 30 minutes inside the fridge before slicing and serving.
**Nutrition Info:**Calories: 118 Carbohydrates: 15 g Fiber: 1 g Fats: 5 g Sodium: 35 mg Protein: 2 g

## Cappuccino Cupcakes

Servings: 17     Cooking Time: 15 Minutes
**Ingredients:**
- 2 eggs
- 2 cups all-purpose flour
- ¼ cup instant coffee granules
- ½ cup of baby food
- ½ cup cocoa, crushed
- What you will need from the store cupboard:
- ¼ cup canola oil
- 1 teaspoon of baking soda
- 2 teaspoons vanilla extract
- ½ teaspoon salt
- 1-1/2 cups low-fat whipped topping
- ½ cup hot water

**Directions:**
Bring together the cocoa, flour, salt, and baking soda in your bowl. Dissolve the coffee granules in hot water. Now whisk together the baby food, eggs, coffee mix, and vanilla in a bowl. Stir the dry ingredients in gradually. Fill into your muffin cups. Bake for 10 to 12 minutes. Sprinkle with cocoa and add the whipped toppings before serving.
**Nutrition Info:**Calories 192, Carbohydrates 33g, Fiber 1g, Sugar 2g, Cholesterol 22mg, Total Fat 5g, Protein 3g

## Quail Eggs & Prosciutto Wraps

Servings: 2     Cooking Time: 10 Minutes
**Ingredients:**
- 3 thin prosciutto slices
- 9 basil leaves
- 9 quail eggs

**Directions:**
Cover the quail eggs with salted water and bring to a boil over medium heat for 2-3 minutes. Place the eggs in an ice bath and let cool for 10 minutes, then peel them. Cut the prosciutto slices into three strips. Place basil leaves at the end of each strip. Top with a quail egg. Wrap in prosciutto, secure with toothpicks and serve.
**Nutrition Info:**Calories 243 Fat: 21g Net Carbs: 0.5g Protein: 12.5g

## Pumpkin Spiced Almonds

Servings: 4     Cooking Time: 25 Minutes
**Ingredients:**
- 1 tablespoon olive oil
- 1 ¼ teaspoon pumpkin pie spice
- Pinch salt
- 1 cup whole almonds, raw

**Directions:**
Preheat the oven to 300°F and line a baking sheet with parchment. Whisk together the olive oil, pumpkin pie spice, and salt in a mixing bowl. Toss in the almonds until evenly coated, then spread on the baking sheet. Bake for 25 minutes then cool completely and store in an airtight container.
**Nutrition Info:**170 calories 15.5g fat 5g protein 5.5g carbs 3g fiber 2.5g net carbs

## Pumpkin Custard

Servings: 6     Cooking Time: 2 Hours 30 Minutes

**Ingredients:**
- 1/2 cup   almond flour
- 4 eggs
- 1 cup pumpkin puree
- 1/2 cup   stevia/erythritol blend, granulated
- 1/8 teaspoon sea salt
- 1 teaspoon vanilla extract or maple flavoring
- 4 tablespoons butter, ghee, or coconut oil melted
- 1 teaspoon pumpkin pie spice

**Directions:**
Grease or spray a slow cooker with butter or coconut oil spray.     In a medium mixing bowl, beat the eggs until smooth. Then add in the sweetener.     To the egg mixture, add in the pumpkin puree along with vanilla or maple extract.     Then add almond flour to the mixture along with the pumpkin pie spice and salt. Add melted butter, coconut oil or ghee.     Transfer the mixture into a slow cooker. Close the lid. Cook for 2-2 ¾ hours on low. When through, serve with whipped cream, and then sprinkle with little nutmeg if need be. Enjoy!     Set slow-cooker to the low setting. Cook for 2-2.45 hours, and begin checking at the two hour mark. Serve warm with stevia sweetened whipped cream and a sprinkle of nutmeg.

**Nutrition Info:**147 calories; 12 g fat; 4 g total carbs; 5 g protein

## Peppers And Hummus

Servings: 4     Cooking Time: 0 Minutes

**Ingredients:**
- one 15-ounce can chickpeas, drained and rinsed
- juice of 1 lemon, or 1 tablespoon lemon juice
- ¼ cup tahini
- 3 tablespoons extra-virgin olive oil
- ½ teaspoon ground cumin
- 1 tablespoon water
- ¼ teaspoon paprika
- 1 red bell pepper, sliced
- 1 green bell pepper, sliced
- 1 orange bell pepper, sliced

**Directions:**
Preparing the Ingredients     In a food processor, combine chickpeas, lemon juice, tahini, 2 tablespoons of the olive oil, the cumin, and water.     Finish and Serve Process on high speed until blended for about 30 seconds. Scoop the hummus into a bowl and drizzle with the remaining tablespoon of olive oil. Sprinkle with paprika and serve with sliced bell peppers.

**Nutrition Info:**Fat: 10 g Protein: 5.4 g Carbohydrates: 22.8 g

## Strawberry Shake

Servings: 2     Cooking Time: 10 Minutes

**Ingredients:**
- 1½ cups fresh strawberries, hulled
- 1 large frozen banana, peeled
- 2 scoops unsweetened vegan vanilla protein powder
- 2 tablespoons hemp seeds
- 2 cups unsweetened hemp milk

**Directions:**
In a high-speed blender, place all the ingredients and pulse until creamy.     Pour into two glasses and serve immediately.

**Nutrition Info:**Calories 325 Total Fat 13 g Saturated Fat 0.8 g Cholesterol 0 mg Sodium 391 mg Total Carbs 23.3 g Fiber 3.9 g Sugar 12.5 g Protein 31.2 g

## Cinnamon Protein Bars

Servings: 8     Cooking Time: 10 Minutes

**Ingredients:**
- 2 scoops vanilla protein powder
- 1/4 cup coconut oil, melted
- 1 cup almond butter
- 1/4 tsp cinnamon
- 12 drops liquid stevia
- Pinch of salt

**Directions:**
In a bowl, mix together all ingredients until well combined.     Transfer bar mixture into a baking dish and press down evenly.     Place in refrigerator until firm. Slice and serve.

**Nutrition Info:**Calories 99 Fat 8 g Carbohydrates 0.6 g Sugar 0.2 g Protein 7.2 g Cholesterol 0 mg

## Chocó Cookies

Servings: 14     Cooking Time: 10 Minutes

**Ingredients:**
- 1 egg
- 1/2 cup erythritol
- 1/4 cup unsweetened cocoa powder
- 1 cup almond butter
- 3 tbsp unsweetened almond milk
- 1/4 cup unsweetened chocolate chips

**Directions:**
Preheat the oven to 350 F/ 180 C.     Line baking tray with parchment paper and set aside.     In a bowl, mix together almond butter, egg, sweetener, almond milk, and cocoa powder until well combined.     Stir in Chocó chips.     Make cookies from mixture and place on a baking tray.     Bake for 10 minutes.     Allow to cool completely then serve.

**Nutrition Info:**Calories 44 Fat 3.5 g Carbohydrates 2.2 g Sugar 0.1 g Protein 1.5 g Cholesterol 12 mg

## Chocolate Avocado Ice Cream

Servings: 6     Cooking Time: 0 Minutes

**Ingredients:**
- Large organic avocados, pitted: 2
- Erythritol, powdered: ½ cup
- Cocoa powder, organic and unsweetened: ½ cup
- Drops of liquid stevia: 25
- Vanilla extract, unsweetened: 2 teaspoons
- Coconut milk, full-fat and unsweetened: 1 cup
- Heavy whipping cream, full-fat: ½ cup
- Squares of chocolate, unsweetened and chopped: 6

**Directions:**

Scoop out the flesh from each avocado, place it in a bowl and add vanilla, milk, and cream and blend using an immersion blender until smooth and creamy. Add remaining ingredients except for chocolate and mix until well combined and smooth. Fold in chopped chocolate and let the mixture chill in the refrigerator for 8 to 12 hours or until cooled. When ready to serve, let ice cream stand for 30 minutes at room temperature, then process it using an ice cream machine as per manufacturer instruction. Serve immediately.

**Nutrition Info:**Calories: 216.7 Fat: 19.4 g Protein: 3.8 g Net Carbs: 3.7 g Fiber: 7.4 g

## Marinated Strawberries

Servings: 6    Cooking Time: 35 Minutes
**Ingredients:**
- 4 cups (2 pints) strawberries
- 1 to 2 tbsps. sugar
- 2 tbsps. aged balsamic vinegar
- 2 tbsps. finely shredded fresh mint
- 1 tbsp. lemon juice
- 3 cups low-fat or fat-free vanilla frozen yogurt

**Directions:**
Cut off strawberry stems; cut strawberries in half or into quarters lengthwise if large. Mix together lemon juice, mint, balsamic vinegar, sugar, and strawberries in a medium bowl. Cover and let chill in the fridge for at least 20 minutes or up to 4 hours. Over scoops of frozen yogurt, spoon the strawberry mixture to serve.

**Nutrition Info:**Calories: 166 calories; Total Carbohydrate: 33 g Cholesterol: 10 mg Total Fat: 2 g Protein: 5 g Sodium: 77 mg Saturated Fat: 1 g

## Tomato & Cheese In Lettuce Packets

Servings: 36    Cooking Time: 15 Minutes
**Ingredients:**
- ¼ pound Gruyere cheese, grated
- ¼ pound feta cheese, crumbled
- ½ tsp oregano
- 1 tomato, chopped
- ½ cup buttermilk
- ½ head lettuce

**Directions:**
In a bowl, mix feta and Gruyere cheese, oregano, tomato, and buttermilk. Separate the lettuce leaves and put them on a serving platter. Divide the mixture between them, roll up, folding in the ends to secure and serve.

**Nutrition Info:**Calories 433 Fat: 32.5g Net Carbs: 6.6g Protein: 27.5g

## Tofu & Chia Seed Pudding

Servings: 4    Cooking Time: 15 Minutes
**Ingredients:**
- 1-pound silken tofu, pressed and drained
- ¼ cup banana, peeled
- 3 tablespoons cacao powder
- 1 teaspoon vanilla extract
- 3 tablespoons chia seeds
- ¼ cup walnuts, chopped
- ¼ cup black raisins

**Directions:**
In a food processor, add tofu, banana, cocoa powder, and vanilla, and pulse till smooth and creamy. Transfer into a large serving bowl and stir in chia seeds till well mixed. Now, place the pudding in serving bowls evenly. With plastic wraps, cover the bowls. Refrigerate to chill before serving. Garnish with raspberries and serve.

**Nutrition Info:**Calories 188 Total Fat 10.4 g Saturated Fat 1.4 g Cholesterol 0 mg Sodium 42 mg Total Carbs 17.1 g Fiber 4.2 g Sugar 8.2 g Protein 12 g

## Mango Mousse

Servings: 6    Cooking Time: 10 Minutes
**Ingredients:**
- 1 banana
- 2 mangoes, seeded, cubed, and peeled
- 2/3 cup plain yogurt
- 1 cup low-fat milk
- 1/8 cup unsweetened coconut
- What you will need from the store cupboard:
- 1 teaspoon vanilla extract
- 6 ice cubes
- 2 teaspoons honey

**Directions:**
Bring together the vanilla extract, yogurt, honey, ice cubes, mangoes and banana in your blender. Blend until it becomes smooth. Refrigerate for a couple of hours. Pour into each dish before serving.

**Nutrition Info:**Calories 87, Carbohydrates 20g, Fiber 2g, Sugar 2g, Cholesterol 1mg, Total Fat 0g, Protein 2g

## Nutty Wild Rice Salad

Servings: 8    Cooking Time: 40 Minutes
**Ingredients:**
- 2/3 cup uncooked wild rice
- cans (14 ounces) sauerkraut rinsed and well drained
- 1 medium apple peeled and chopped
- 3/4 cup celery chopped
- 3/4 cup carrot shredded (about 1 large carrot)
- 1/2 cup red onion finely chopped
- Dressing
- 1/2 cup sugar
- 1/3 cup cider vinegar
- 1 tbsp canola oil
- 1/4 tsp salt
- 1/4 tsp pepper
- 1 tbsp fresh parsley minced
- 1 tbsp fresh tarragon minced (or 1 tsp dried tarragon)
- 3/4 cup walnuts chopped, toasted

**Directions:**
Cook wild rice according to package directions. Cool completely. In a large bowl, combine sauerkraut, apple, celery, carrot, onion and cooled rice. In a small bowl, whisk the first five dressing ingredients until sugar is dissolved; stir in herbs. Add to sauerkraut mixture; toss to combine. Refrigerate, covered, at least 4 hours to allow flavours to blend. Stir in walnuts just before serving. Tip: To toast nuts, bake in a shallow pan in a

350° oven for 5-10 minutes or cook in a skillet over low heat until lightly browned, stirring occasionally.
**Nutrition Info:**300 calories 27.5g fat 6g protein 14.5g carbs 10g fiber 4.5g net carbs

## Banana Split Sundae

Servings: 4    Cooking Time: 0 Minutes
**Ingredients:**
- 3 frozen, sliced overripe bananas (see Tip)
- 2 tbsps. peanut butter
- 1 tbsp. thawed frozen light whipped topping
- 1 tsp. sugar-free chocolate-flavor syrup
- 1 tsp. chopped peanuts
- 1 maraschino cherry

**Directions:**
Combine peanut butter and bananas in a food processor. Process with cover until almost no lumps remain. Scoop the mixture into sundae dishes.    Garnish top with whipped topping, maraschino cherry, peanuts and sugar-free chocolate-flavor syrup. Serve right away.
**Nutrition Info:**Calories: 166 calories Total Carbohydrate: 27 g Cholesterol: 0 mg Total Fat: 6 g Fiber: 3 g Protein: 3 g Sodium: 60 mg Sugar: 14 g Saturated Fat: 2 g

## Tzatziki Dip With Cauliflower

Servings: 6    Cooking Time: 0 Minutes
**Ingredients:**
- ½ (8-ounce) package cream cheese, softened
- 1 cup sour cream
- 1 tablespoon ranch seasoning
- 1 English cucumber, diced
- 2 tablespoons chopped chives
- 2 cups cauliflower florets

**Directions:**
Beat the cream cheese with an electric mixer until creamy.    Add the sour cream and ranch seasoning, then beat until smooth.    Fold in the cucumbers and chives, then chill before serving with cauliflower florets for dipping.
**Nutrition Info:**125 calories 10.5g fat 3g protein 5.5g carbs 1g fiber 4.5g net carbs

## Plum & Pistachio Snack

Servings: 1    Cooking Time: 5 Minutes
**Ingredients:**
- ¼ cup unsalted dry-roasted pistachios (measured in shell)
- 1 plum

**Directions:**
Hull and serve pistachios together with plum.
**Nutrition Info:**Calories: 113 calories; Total Carbohydrate: 12 g Cholesterol: 0 mg Total Fat: 7 g Fiber: 2 g Protein: 4 g Sodium: 1 mg Sugar: 8 g Saturated Fat: 1 g

## Fruity Tofu Smoothie

Servings: 2    Cooking Time: 10 Minutes
**Ingredients:**
- 12 ounces' silken tofu, pressed and drained

- 2 medium bananas, peeled
- 1½ cups fresh blueberries
- 1 tablespoon maple syrup
- 1½ cups unsweetened soymilk
- ¼ cup ice cubes

**Directions:**
Place all the ingredients in a high-speed blender and pulse until creamy.    Pour into two glasses and serve immediately.
**Nutrition Info:**Calories 398 Total Fat 8.6 g Saturated Fat 1.2 g Cholesterol 0 mg Sodium 58 mg Total Carbs 65 g Fiber 7 g Sugar 50.7 g Protein 19.9 g

## Strawberry Mousse

Servings: 6
**Ingredients:**
- 1½ cups fresh strawberries, hulled
- 1 2/3 cups chilled unsweetened almond milk
- 2-3 drops liquid stevia
- 1 teaspoon organic vanilla extract

**Directions:**
In a food processor, add all the ingredients and pulse until smooth.    Transfer into serving bowls and serve. Meal Prep Tip: Transfer the mousse into an airtight container. Cover the containers and refrigerate for up to 3 days.
**Nutrition Info:**Calories 25 Total Fat 1.1g Saturated Fat 0.1 g Cholesterol 0 mg Total Carbs 3.4 g Sugar 1.9 g Fiber 1 g Sodium 50 mg Potassium 109 mg Protein 0.5 g

## Raisin Apple Cake

Servings: 6    Cooking Time: 10 Minutes
**Ingredients:**
- 2 eggs, beaten
- ½ cup raisins
- ½ cup whole-wheat flour
- 1 cup all-purpose flour
- 1 teaspoon cinnamon, ground
- What you will need from the store cupboard:
- 2 teaspoons baking powder
- 1 cup applesauce
- 2 teaspoons vanilla extract

**Directions:**
Bring together the eggs, apple sauce, cinnamon, flour, baking powder, vanilla and raisins in your mixing bowl. Use the batter to make small cakes.    Now heat your girdle on medium heat.    Fry the cakes. Make sure that both sides are brown.
**Nutrition Info:**Calories 203, Carbohydrates 41g, Fiber 3g, Sugar 1.4g, Cholesterol 62mg, Total Fat 1g, Protein 6g

## Avocado And Tempeh Bacon Wraps

Servings: 4    Cooking Time: 8 Minutes
**Ingredients:**
- 2 tablespoons extra-virgin olive oil
- 8 ounces tempeh bacon, homemade or store-bought
- 4 (10-inch) soft flour tortillas or lavish flat bread

- ¼ cup vegan mayonnaise, homemade or store-bought
- 4 large lettuce leaves
- 2 ripe Hass avocados, pitted, peeled, and cut into ¼-inch slices
- 1 large ripe tomato, cut into ¼-inch slices

**Directions:**
Preparing the Ingredients    Cook the tempeh bacon until browned on both sides in a large skillet about 8 minutes. Remove from the heat and set aside.    Place 1 tortilla on a work surface. Spread with some of the mayonnaise and one-fourth of the lettuce and tomatoes. Finish and Serve    Pit, peel, and thinly slice the avocado and place the slices on top of the tomato. Add the reserved tempeh bacon and roll up tightly. Repeat with remaining Ingredients and serve.

**Nutrition Info:** Fat: 24.3 g Protein: 11.7 g Carbohydrates: 16.7 g

## Coco-macadamia Fat Bombs

Servings: 16    Cooking Time: 0 Minutes
**Ingredients:**
- 1 cup coconut oil
- 1 cup smooth almond butter
- ½ cup unsweetened cocoa powder
- ¼ cup coconut flour
- Liquid stevia extract, to taste
- 16 whole macadamia nuts, raw

**Directions:**
Melt the coconut oil and cashew butter together in a small saucepan.    Whisk in the cocoa powder, coconut flour, and liquid stevia to taste.    Remove from heat and let cool until it hardens slightly.    Divide the mixture into 16 even pieces.    Roll each piece into a ball around a macadamia nut and chill until ready to eat.

**Nutrition Info:** 255 calories 25.5g fat 3.5g protein 7g carbs 3g fiber 4g net carbs

## Chocolate-covered Prosecco Strawberries

Servings: 2    Cooking Time: 45 Minutes
**Ingredients:**
- 12 medium strawberries, rinsed and dried
- 2 cups prosecco or other sparkling wine
- ⅓ cup bittersweet chocolate chips (2 oz.)

**Directions:**
In a medium bowl, combine prosecco and strawberries. Keep the strawberries submerged by placing a bowl on top. Cover and place in the refrigerator overnight or for at least 8 hours.    Transfer the strawberries to a plate lined with paper towels and pat dry. In a microwave-safe bowl, put the chocolate chips. Microwave in 20-second intervals on High, stirring each interval, until chocolate is melted, about 1 minute. Dip strawberries into the chocolate and put them onto a plate lined with waxed paper. Let sit in refrigerator until the chocolate is firm, about 15 to 20 minutes.

**Nutrition Info:** Calories: 50 calories; Total Carbohydrate: 7 g Cholesterol: 0 mg Total Fat: 3 g Fiber: 1 g Protein: 1 g Sodium: 0 mg Sugar: 5 g Saturated Fat: 1 g

## Pumpkin Spice Snack Balls

Servings: 10    Cooking Time: 10 Minutes
**Ingredients:**
- 1 ½ cups old-fashioned oats
- ½ cup chopped almonds
- ½ cup unsweetened shredded coconut
- ¾ cup canned pumpkin puree
- 2 tablespoons honey
- 2 teaspoons pumpkin pie spice
- ¼ teaspoon salt

**Directions:**
Preheat the oven to 300°F and line a baking sheet with parchment.    Combine the oats, almonds, and coconut on the baking sheet.    Bake for 8 to 10 minutes until browned, stirring halfway through.    Place the pumpkin, honey, pumpkin pie spice, and salt in a medium bowl.    Stir in the toasted oat mixture. Shape the mixture into 20 balls by hand and place on a tray.    Chill until the balls are firm then serve.

**Nutrition Info:** Calories 170, Total Fat 9.8g, Saturated Fat 6g, Total Carbs 17.8g, Net Carbs 13.7g, Protein 3.8g, Sugar 5.2g, Fiber 4.1g, Sodium 64mg

## Chocolatey Banana Shake

Servings: 2    Cooking Time: 10 Minutes
**Ingredients:**
- 2 medium frozen bananas, peeled
- 4 dates, pitted
- 4 tablespoons peanut butter
- 4 tablespoons rolled oats
- 2 tablespoons cacao powder
- 2 tablespoons chia seeds
- 2 cups unsweetened soymilk

**Directions:**
Place all the ingredients in a high-speed blender and pulse until creamy.    Pour into two glasses and serve immediately.

**Nutrition Info:** Calories 583 Total Fat 25.2 g Saturated Fat 4.8 g Cholesterol 0 mg Sodium 200 mg Total Carbs 75 g Fiber 15.3 g Sugar 37.8 g Protein 23.1 g

## Chia Strawberry Pudding

Servings: 4    Cooking Time: 10 Minutes
**Ingredients:**
- 1 tsp unsweetened cocoa powder
- 5 tbsp chia seeds
- 2 tbsp xylitol
- 1 1/2 tsp vanilla
- 1 ½ cups strawberries, chopped
- 1 cup unsweetened coconut milk
- Pinch of salt

**Directions:**
In a saucepan, combine together strawberries, ½ cup water, xylitol, vanilla, and salt and simmer over medium heat for 5-10 minutes.    Mash strawberries with a fork. Add coconut milk and stir to combine.    Add chia seeds and mix well and let it sit for 5 minutes.    Pour pudding mixture in serving glasses.    Sprinkle cocoa powder on top of chia pudding.    Place in refrigerator for 1 hour. Serve chilled and enjoy.

**Nutrition Info:**Calories 211 Fat 17.4 g Carbohydrates 11 g Sugar 4.9 g Protein 3.8 g Cholesterol 0 mg

## Chocolate Banana Cake

Servings: 12    Cooking Time: 20 Minutes
**Ingredients:**
- 2 eggs
- 1 cup ripe bananas, mashed
- 1-1/3 cups all-purpose flour
- 3 tablespoons cocoa, crushed
- 1 cup low-fat milk
- What you will need from the store cupboard:
- 2 teaspoons vanilla extract
- ½ teaspoon baking soda
- 1 teaspoon baking powder
- 1/3 cup butter
- ½ teaspoon salt
- ½ cup of water
- Cooking spray

**Directions:**
Preheat your oven to 350 °F. Apply cooking spray to your baking pan.    Add butter until it is fluffy and light. Add the eggs and vanilla (1 at a time). Beat after each addition.    Now stir the water in.    Whisk together the milk, flour, baking powder, cocoa, salt, and baking soda. Add this to the creamed mix. Combine well.    Stir the bananas in.    Place in your pan and bake.
**Nutrition Info:**Calories 169, Carbohydrates 25g, Fiber 1g, Sugar 1g, Cholesterol 45mg, Total Fat 6g, Protein 4g

## Delicious Egg Cups With Cheese & Spinach

Servings: 2    Cooking Time: 10 Minutes
**Ingredients:**
- 4 eggs
- 1 tbsp fresh parsley, chopped
- ¼ cup cheddar cheese, shredded
- ¼ cup spinach, chopped
- Salt and black pepper to taste

**Directions:**
Grease muffin cups with cooking spray. In a bowl, whisk the eggs and add in the rest of the ingredients. Season with salt and black pepper. Fill ¾ parts of each muffin cup with the egg mixture.    Bake in the oven for 15 minutes at 390 F. Serve warm!
**Nutrition Info:**Calories: 232 Fat 14.3g Net Carbs 1.5g Protein 16.2g

## Lemon Custard

Servings: 4    Cooking Time: 3 Hours
**Ingredients:**
- 2 cups whipping cream or coconut cream
- 5 egg yolks
- 1 tablespoon lemon zest
- 1 teaspoon vanilla extract
- 1/4 cup fresh lemon juice, squeezed
- 1/2 teaspoon liquid stevia
- Lightly sweetened whipped cream

**Directions:**

Whisk egg yolks together with lemon zest, liquid stevia, lemon zest and vanilla in a bowl, and then whisk in heavy cream.    Divide the mixture among 4 small jars or ramekins.    To the bottom of a slow cooker add a rack, and then add ramekins on top of the rack and add enough water to cover half of ramekins.    Close the lid and cook for 3 hours on low. Remove ramekins.    Let cool to room temperature, and then place into the refrigerator to cool completely for about 3 hours. When through, top with the whipped cream and serve. Enjoy!
**Nutrition Info:**319 calories; 30 g fat; 3 g total carbs; 7 g protein

## Yogurt Cheesecake

Servings: 8    Cooking Time: 35 Minutes
**Ingredients:**
- 2½ cups fat-free plain Greek yogurt
- 6-8 drops liquid stevia
- 3 egg whites
- 1/3 cup cacao powder
- ¼ cup arrowroot starch
- 1 teaspoon organic vanilla extract
- Pinch of sea salt

**Directions:**
Preheat the oven to 35 degrees F. Grease a 9-inch cake pan.    In a large bowl, add all ingredients and mix until well combined.    Place the mixture into the prepared pan evenly.    Bake for about 30-35 minutes. Remove from oven and let it cool completely. Refrigerate to chill for about 3-4 hours or until set completely.    Cut into 8 equal sized slices and serve. Meal Prep Tip: With foil pieces, wrap the cheesecake slices and refrigerate for about 1-3 days. Reheat in the microwave before serving.
**Nutrition Info:**Calories 74 Total Fat 0.9g Saturated Fat 0.4 g Cholesterol 2 mg Total Carbs 8.5 g Sugar 3 g Fiber 1.1 g Sodium 89 mg Potassium 21 mg Protein 9.5 g

## Fruit Salad

Servings: 6    Cooking Time: 0 Minute
**Ingredients:**
- 8 oz. light cream cheese
- 6 oz. Greek yogurt
- 1 tablespoon honey
- 1 teaspoon orange zest
- 1 teaspoon lemon zest
- 1 orange, sliced into sections
- 3 kiwi fruit, peeled and sliced
- 1 mango, cubed
- 1 cup blueberries

**Directions:**
Beat cream cheese using an electric mixer.    Add yogurt and honey.    Beat until smooth.    Stir in the orange and lemon zest.    Toss the fruits to mix.    Divide in glass jars.    Top with the cream cheese mixture.
**Nutrition Info:**Calories 131 Total Fat 3 g Saturated Fat 2 g Cholesterol 9 mg Sodium 102 mg Total Carbohydrate 23 g Dietary Fiber 3 g Total Sugars 18 g Protein 5 g Potassium 234 mg

## Risotto Bites

Servings: 12    Cooking Time: 20 Minutes

**Ingredients:**
- ½ cup panko bread crumbs
- 1 teaspoon paprika
- 1 teaspoon chipotle powder or ground cayenne pepper
- 1½ cups cold Green Pea Risotto
- Nonstick cooking spray

**Directions:**

Preparing the Ingredients    Preheat the oven to 425°F. Line a baking sheet with parchment paper.    On a large plate, combine the panko, paprika, and chipotle powder. Set aside.    Roll 2 tablespoons of the risotto into a ball. Gently roll in the bread crumbs, and place on the prepared baking sheet. Repeat to make a total of 12 balls. Bake    Spritz the tops of the risotto bites with nonstick cooking spray and bake for 15-20 minutes until they begin to brown.    Finish and Serve    Cool completely before storing in a large airtight container in a single layer (add a piece of parchment paper for a second layer), or in a plastic freezer bag.

**Nutrition Info:** Calories: 100 Fat: 2g Protein: 6g Carbohydrates: 17g Fiber: 5g Sugar: 2g Sodium: 165mg

# Other Favorite Recipes

## Grilled Avocado Hummus Paninis

Servings: 4    Cooking Time: 10 Minutes
**Ingredients:**
- 4 whole-wheat sandwich thins, split in half
- 1/3 cup roasted red pepper hummus
- ½ medium avocado, pitted and sliced thin
- Fresh ground pepper
- 1 cup fresh baby spinach, chopped
- 2 ounces feta cheese

**Directions:**
Lay the sandwich thins out flat.    Spread the hummus evenly on both sides of each sandwich thin.    Layer the avocado slices on the bottom of each sandwich thin and season with fresh ground black pepper.    Top each sandwich with ¼ cup spinach and ½ ounce cheese. Add the top to each sandwich and press down lightly. Grease a large skillet with cooking spray and heat over medium heat.    Add one or two sandwiches and place a heavy skillet on top.    Cook for 2 minutes or until the bottoms are toasted.    Flip the sandwiches and repeat on the other side. Cut in half to serve.
**Nutrition Info:**Calories 230, Total Fat 11.2g, Saturated Fat 3.2g, Total Carbs 27.8g, Net Carbs 19.2g, Protein 8.5g, Sugar 3.5g, Fiber 8.6g, Sodium 508mg

## Cauliflower Muffin

Servings: 4    Cooking Time: 30 Minutes
**Ingredients:**
- 2,5 cup cauliflower
- 2/3 cup ham
- 2,5 cups of cheese
- 2/3 cup champignon
- 1,5 tbsp. flaxseed
- 3 eggs
- 1/4 tsp. salt
- 1/8 tsp. pepper

**Directions:**
Preheat oven to 375 F.    Put muffin liners in a 12-muffin tin.    Combine diced cauliflower, ground flaxseed, beaten eggs, cup diced ham, grated cheese, and diced mushrooms, salt, pepper.    Divide mixture rightly between muffin liners.    Bake 30 Minutes.    This is a great lunch for the whole family.
**Nutrition Info:**Calories 116 / Protein 10 g / Fat 7 g / Carbs 3 g

## Bok Choy Soup

Servings: 4    Cooking Time: 25 Minutes
**Ingredients:**
- 2 tablespoons coconut oil, melted
- 1-pound bok choy, torn
- 2 shallots, chopped
- 4 cups chicken stock
- 1 cup heavy cream
- 1 tablespoon cilantro, chopped
- A pinch of salt and black pepper

- ½ teaspoon nutmeg, ground

**Directions:**
Heat up a pot with the oil over medium heat, add the shallots and sauté for 5 minutes.    Add the bok choy and the other ingredients, bring to a simmer and cook over medium heat for 20 minutes.    Blend the soup using an immersion blender, divide into bowls and serve.
**Nutrition Info:**calories 194 fat 18.4 fiber 1.4 carbs 5.4 protein 3.2

## Stuffed Mushrooms

Servings: 4    Cooking Time: 20 Minutes
**Ingredients:**
- 4 Portobello Mushrooms, large
- 1/2 cup Mozzarella Cheese, shredded
- 1/2 cup Marinara, low-sugar
- Olive Oil Spray

**Directions:**
Preheat the oven to 375 F.    Take out the dark gills from the mushrooms with the help of a spoon.    Keep the mushroom stem upside down and spoon it with two tablespoons of marinara sauce and mozzarella cheese. Bake for 18 minutes or until the cheese is bubbly.
**Nutrition Info:**Calories – 113kL; Fat – 6g; Carbohydrates – 4g; Protein – 7g; Sodium – 14mg

## Roasted Salmon With Lemon

Servings: 6    Cooking Time: 25 Minutes
**Ingredients:**
- 1 salmon whole-side fillet, skin on
- 2 T. lemon juice
- 1 bunch fresh dill, chopped
- 4 T. butter
- 2 T. white wine
- 1/2 tsp. kosher salt
- 1/4 tsp. freshly ground black pepper

**Directions:**
Allow salmon to come to room temperature before baking. Preheat oven to 425°F. Mix dill and lemon juice in a small bowl. Lay fillet skin-side down on a parchment-lined baking sheet and cover with lemon-dill mixture. Top with butter, white wine, salt, and pepper. Bake uncovered until the fish flakes easily with a fork, about 20-25 minutes.
**Nutrition Info:**Calories: 146.7    Fat: 10.9g Cholesterol: 49.1mg    Sodium: 237.3mg    Potassium: 269.5mg    Carbohydrates: 0.8g    Dietary Fiber: 0.1g Sugars: 0.2g    Protein: 10.3g

## White Spinach Pizza With Cauliflower Crust

Servings: 1 10-inch Pizza    Cooking Time: 25 Minutes
**Ingredients:**
- 1 head cauliflower, trimmed and chopped
- 2 eggs, beaten
- 2 c. shredded mozzarella cheese, divided
- 1/4 c. grated Parmesan cheese
- 2 tsp. Italian seasoning

- 3 T. extra virgin olive oil
- 1/2 c. shredded provolone cheese
- 3/4 c. whole milk ricotta cheese
- 3 cloves garlic, minced
- 1/4 c. thinly sliced red onion
- 1 c. baby spinach, washed

**Directions:**
To make the crust, pulse cauliflower florets in a food processor until they resemble rice. Microwave, covered loosely, for 5 minutes. Drain cauliflower in paper towel or cheesecloth, wringing out the towel to remove as much moisture as possible. Mix drained cauliflower with eggs, 1/2 cup of the mozzarella, Parmesan, and Italian seasoning. Press into a 10-inch round (or 10x15-inch rectangle) and bake at 425°F for 10-15 minutes. Brush crust with olive oil and top with remaining mozzarella, provolone, ricotta, garlic, red onion, and spinach. Bake for an additional 10 minutes or until the cheese is melted. This crust recipe will work with any toppings.
**Nutrition Info:**Calories: 350.3   Fat: 25.6g   Cholesterol: 116.7mg   Sodium: 558.7mg   Potassium: 415.8mg   Carbohydrates: 9.3g   Dietary Fiber: 2.8g   Sugars: 0.8g   Protein: 22.4g

## Chickpea, Tuna, And Kale Salad

Servings: 1      Cooking Time: None
**Ingredients:**
- 2 ounces fresh kale
- 2 tablespoons fat-free honey mustard dressing
- 1 (3-ounce) pouch tuna in water, drained
- 1 medium carrot, shredded
- Salt and pepper

**Directions:**
Trim the thick stems from the kale and cut into bite-sized pieces.   Toss the kale with the dressing in a salad bowl. Top with tuna, chickpeas, and carrots. Season with salt and pepper to serve.
**Nutrition Info:**Calories 215, Total Fat 0.6g, Saturated Fat 0g, Total Carbs 28.1g, Net Carbs 23.6g, Protein 22.5g, Sugar 16g, Fiber 4.5g, Sodium 1176mg

## Tomato Risotto

Servings: 4      Cooking Time: 30 Minutes
**Ingredients:**
- 1 cup shallots, chopped
- cups cauliflower rice
- tablespoons olive oil
- cups veggie stock
- 1 cup tomatoes, crushed
- 1/4 cup cilantro, chopped
- 1/2 teaspoon chili powder
- 1 teaspoon cumin, ground
- 1 teaspoon coriander, ground

**Directions:**
Heat up a pan with the oil over medium heat, add the shallots and sauté for 5 minutes.    Add the cauliflower rice, tomatoes and the other ingredients, toss, cook over medium heat for 25 minutes more, divide between plates and serve.
**Nutrition Info:**Calories 200 Fat 4 Fiber 3 Carbs 6 Protein 8

## Oats Coffee Smoothie

Servings: 2      Cooking Time: 5 Minutes
**Ingredients:**
- 1 cup Oats, uncooked & grounded
- 2 tbsp. Instant Coffee
- 3 cup Milk, skimmed
- 2 Banana, frozen & sliced into chunks
- 2 tbsp. Flax Seeds, grounded

**Directions:**
Place all of the ingredients in a high-speed blender and blend for 2 minutes or until smooth and luscious. Serve and enjoy.
**Nutrition Info:**Calories: 251Kcal; Carbs 10.9g; Proteins: 20.3g; Fat: 15.1g; Sodium: 102mg

## Premium Roasted Baby Potatoes

Servings: 4      Cooking Time: 35 Minutes
**Ingredients:**
- 2 pounds' new yellow potatoes, scrubbed and cut into wedges
- 2 tablespoons extra virgin olive oil
- 2 teaspoons fresh rosemary, chopped
- 1 teaspoon garlic powder
- 1 teaspoon sweet paprika
- 1/2 teaspoon sea salt
- 1/2 teaspoon freshly ground black pepper

**Directions:**
Pre-heat your oven to 400 degrees Fahrenheit.     Line baking sheet with aluminum foil and set it aside.     Take a large bowl and add potatoes, olive oil, garlic, rosemary, paprika, sea salt and pepper.     Spread potatoes in single layer on baking sheet and bake for 35 minutes. Serve and enjoy!
**Nutrition Info:**Calories: 225 Fat: 7g Carbohydrates: 37g Protein: 5g

## Chicken, Strawberry, And Avocado Salad

Cooking Time: 5 Minutes
**Ingredients:**
- 1,5 cups chicken (skin removed)
- 1/4 cup almonds
- 2 (5-oz) pkg salad greens
- 1 (16-oz) pkg strawberries
- 1 avocado
- 1/4 cup green onion
- 1/4 cup lime juice
- 3 tbsp. extra virgin olive oil
- 2 tbsp. honey
- 1/4 tsp. salt
- 1/4 tsp. pepper

**Directions:**
Toast almonds until golden and fragrant.    Mix lime juice, oil, honey, salt, and pepper.    Mix greens, sliced strawberries, chicken, diced avocado, and sliced green onion and sliced almonds; drizzle with dressing. Toss to coat.    Yummy!
**Nutrition Info:**Calories 150 / Protein 15 g / Fat 10 g / Carbs 5 g

- Salt and pepper

**Directions:**
Heat the oil in a large skillet over medium-high heat. Add the garlic and cook for 1 minute. Stir in the spinach and season with salt and pepper. Sauté for 1 to 2 minutes until just wilted. Serve hot.

**Nutrition Info:** Calories 60, Total Fat 5.5g, Saturated Fat 0.8g, Total Carbs 2.6g, Net Carbs 1.5g, Protein 1.5g, Sugar 0.2g, Fiber 1.1g, Sodium 36mg

## Garlic Bread

Servings: 4-5     Cooking Time: 15 Minutes

**Ingredients:**
- 2 stale French rolls
- 4 tbsp. crushed or crumpled garlic
- 1 cup of mayonnaise
- Powdered grated Parmesan
- 1 tbsp. olive oil

**Directions:**
Preheat the air fryer. Set the time of 5 minutes and the temperature to 2000C. Mix mayonnaise with garlic and set aside. Cut the baguettes into slices, but without separating them completely. Fill the cavities of equals. Brush with olive oil and sprinkle with grated cheese. Place in the basket of the air fryer. Set the timer to 10 minutes, adjust the temperature to 1800C and press the power button.

**Nutrition Info:** Calories: 340 Fat: 15g Carbohydrates: 32g Protein: 15g Sugar: 0g Cholesterol: 0mg

## Tuna Avocado Salad

Servings: 4     Cooking Time: 0 Minutes

**Ingredients:**
- 1 avocado, pit removed and sliced
- 1 lemon, juiced
- 1 tablespoon chopped onion
- 5 ounces cooked or canned tuna
- Salt and pepper to taste

**Directions:**
In a mixing bowl, combine the avocado and lime juice. Mash the avocado and add the tuna. Season with salt and pepper to taste. Serve chilled.

**Nutrition Info:** Calories: 695.5g Fat: 50.7 g Protein: 41.5 g Carbs: 18.3 g

## French Toast In Sticks

Servings: 4     Cooking Time: 10 Minutes

**Ingredients:**
- 4 slices of white bread, 38 mm thick, preferably hard
- 2 eggs
- 60 ml of milk
- 15 ml maple sauce
- 2 ml vanilla extract
- Nonstick Spray Oil
- 38g of sugar
- 3ground cinnamon
- Maple syrup, to serve
- Sugar to sprinkle

**Directions:**

Cut each slice of bread into thirds making 12 pieces. Place sideways     Beat the eggs, milk, maple syrup and vanilla. Preheat the air fryer, set it to 175C.     Dip the sliced bread in the egg mixture and place it in the preheated air fryer. Sprinkle French toast generously with oil spray. Cook French toast for 10 minutes at 175C. Turn the toast halfway through cooking.     Mix the sugar and cinnamon in a bowl.     Cover the French toast with the sugar and cinnamon mixture when you have finished cooking.     Serve with Maple syrup and sprinkle with powdered sugar

**Nutrition Info:** Calories 128 Fat 6.2 g, Carbohydrates 16.3 g, Sugar 3.3 g, Protein 3.2 g, Cholesterol 17 mg

## Strawberry Salsa

Servings: 4     Cooking Time: 5 Minutes;

**Ingredients:**
- 4 tomatoes, seeded and chopped
- 1-pint strawberry, chopped
- 1 red onion, chopped
- 2 tablespoons of juice from a lime
- 1 jalapeno pepper, minced
- What you will need from the store cupboard:
- 1 tablespoon olive oil
- 2 garlic cloves, minced

**Directions:**
Bring together the strawberries, tomatoes, jalapeno, and onion in the bowl. Stir in the garlic, oil, and lime juice. Refrigerate. Serve with separately cooked pork or poultry.

**Nutrition Info:** Calories 19, Carbs 3g, Fiber 1g, Sugar 0.2g, Cholesterol 0mg, Total Fat 1g, Protein 0g

## Southwestern Bean-and-pepper Salad

Servings: 4     Cooking Time: 0 Minutes

**Ingredients:**
- 1 (15-ounce) can pinto beans, drained and rinsed
- 2 bell peppers, cored and chopped
- 1 cup corn kernels (cut from 1 to 2 ears or frozen and thawed)
- Salt
- Freshly ground black pepper
- Juice of 2 limes
- 1 tablespoon olive oil
- 1 avocado, chopped

**Directions:**
In a large bowl, combine beans, peppers, corn, salt, and pepper. Squeeze fresh lime juice to taste and stir in olive oil. Let the mixture stand in the refrigerator for 30 minutes.     Add avocado just before serving. Budget-saver tip avocado prices can vary dramatically depending on their availability. In addition, while avocado in your salad can really add flavor and satiety, for an equally delicious salad you could add a cup of cooked and chopped sweet potatoes with 1 to 2 tablespoons of sunflower seeds.

**Nutrition Info:** Total calories: 245 Total fat: 11g Saturated fat: 2g Cholesterol: 0mg Sodium: 97mg Potassium: 380mg Total carbohydrate: 32g Fiber: 10g Sugars: 4g Protein: 8g.

## Sautéed Turkey Bowl

Servings: 1    Cooking Time: 10 Minutes
**Ingredients:**
- 4 ounces boneless, skinless turkey breast
- 1 teaspoon olive oil
- 1 ½ teaspoons balsamic vinegar
- ½ teaspoon dried basil
- ¼ teaspoon dried thyme
- Salt and pepper
- ¼ cup instant brown rice

**Directions:**
Toss the turkey with the olive oil, balsamic vinegar, basil, and thyme.    Season lightly with salt and pepper then cover and chill for 20 minutes.    Bring ¼ cup of water to boil in a small saucepan.    Stir in the brown rice then simmer for 5 minutes and remove from heat, covered. Meanwhile, heat a small skillet over medium heat and grease lightly with cooking spray.    Add the marinated turkey and sauté for 6 to 8 minutes until cooked through. Spoon the turkey over the brown rice and serve hot.
**Nutrition Info:**Calories 200, Total Fat 6.8g, Saturated Fat 1.1g, Total Carbs 13.3g, Net Carbs 12.1g, Protein 20.4g, Sugar 4g, Fiber 1.2g, Sodium 1152mg

## Cauliflower & Apple Salad

Servings: 4    Cooking Time: 0 Minutes
**Ingredients:**
- 3 Cups Cauliflower, Chopped into Florets
- 2 Cups Baby Kale
- 1 Sweet Apple, Cored & Chopped
- ¼ Cup Basil, Fresh & Chopped
- ¼ Cup Mint, Fresh & Chopped
- ¼ Cup Parsley, Fresh & Chopped
- 1/3 Cup Scallions, Sliced Thin
- 2 Tablespoons Yellow Raisins
- 1 Tablespoon Sun Dried Tomatoes, Chopped
- ½ Cup Miso Dressing, Optional
- ¼ Cup Roasted Pumpkin Seeds, Optional

**Directions:**
Combine everything together, tossing before serving. Interesting Facts: This vegetable is an extremely high source of vitamin A, vitamin B1, B2 and B3.
**Nutrition Info:**Calories: 198 Protein: 7 Grams Fat: 8 Grams Carbs: 32 Grams

## Zucchini Risotto

Servings: 4    Cooking Time: 30 Minutes
**Ingredients:**
- ½ cup shallots, chopped
- tablespoons olive oil
- garlic cloves, minced
- cups cauliflower rice
- cup zucchinis, cubed
- cups veggie stock
- ½ cup white mushrooms, chopped
- ½ teaspoon coriander, ground
- A pinch of salt and black pepper
- ¼ teaspoon oregano, dried
- tablespoons parsley, chopped

**Directions:**
Heat up a pan with the oil over medium heat, add the shallots, garlic, mushrooms, coriander and oregano, stir

and sauté for 10 minutes.    Add the cauliflower rice and the other ingredients, toss, cook for 20 minutes more, divide between plates and serve.
**Nutrition Info:**Calories 231 fat 5 fiber 3 carbs 9 protein 12

## Peanut Butter Mousse

Servings: 2    Cooking Time: 10 Minutes
**Ingredients:**
- 1 tbsp. peanut butter
- 1 tsp. vanilla extract
- 1 tsp. stevia
- 1/2 cup heavy cream

**Directions:**
Add all ingredients into the bowl and whisk until soft peak forms.    Spoon into the serving bowls and enjoy.
**Nutrition Info:**Calories 157 Fat 15.1 g, Carbohydrates 5.2 g, Sugar 3.6 g, Protein 2.6 g, Cholesterol 41 mg

## Peanut Butter Banana Smoothie

Servings: 1    Cooking Time: 2 Minutes
**Ingredients:**
- ¼ cup Greek Yoghurt, plain
- 1/2 tbsp. Chia Seeds
- 1/2 cup Ice Cubes
- 1/2 of 1 Banana
- 1/2 cup Water
- 1 tbsp. Peanut Butter

**Directions:**
Place all the ingredients needed to make the smoothie in a high-speed blender and blend to get a smooth and luscious mixture.    Transfer the smoothie to a serving glass and enjoy it.
**Nutrition Info:**Calories: 202cal; Carbohydrates: 14g; Proteins: 10g; Fat: 9g; Sodium: 30mg

## Salmon With Asparagus

Servings: 3    Cooking Time: 10 Minutes
**Ingredients:**
- 1 lb. Salmon, sliced into fillets
- 1 tbsp. Olive Oil
- Salt & Pepper, as needed
- 1 bunch of Asparagus, trimmed
- 2 cloves of Garlic, minced
- Zest & Juice of 1/2 Lemon
- 1 tbsp. Butter, salted

**Directions:**
Spoon in the butter and olive oil into a large pan and heat it over medium-high heat.    Once it becomes hot, place the salmon and season it with salt and pepper.    Cook for 4 minutes per side and then cook the other side. Stir in the garlic and lemon zest to it.    Cook for further 2 minutes or until slightly browned.    Off the heat and squeeze the lemon juice over it.    Serve it hot.
**Nutrition Info:**Calories: 409Kcal; Carbohydrates: 2.7g; Proteins: 32.8g; Fat: 28.8g; Sodium: 497mg

## Roasted Tomatoes

Servings: 4    Cooking Time: 25 Minutes
**Ingredients:**
- 1-pound tomatoes, halved
- A pinch of salt and black pepper
- 2 tablespoons olive oil
- 1 teaspoon rosemary, dried
- 1 teaspoon basil, dried

112

- 1 tablespoon chives, chopped

**Directions:**
In a roasting pan combine the tomatoes with the oil and the other ingredients, toss gently and bake at 390 degrees F for 25 minutes. Divide the mix between plates and serve.
**Nutrition Info:**calories 124 fat 14 fiber 4 carbs 4 protein 14

## Crispy Radishes

Servings: 4    Cooking Time: 20 Minutes
**Ingredients:**
- Cooking spray
- 15 radishes, sliced
- Salt and black pepper to the taste
- 1 tablespoon chives, chopped

**Directions:**
Arrange radish slices on a lined baking sheet and spray them with cooking oil. Season with salt and pepper and sprinkle chives, introduce in the oven at 375 degrees F and bake for 10 minutes. Flip them and bake for 10 minutes more. Serve them cold. Enjoy!
**Nutrition Info:**calories 34 fat 4 fiber 0.4 carbs 4 protein 0.1

## Edamame Salad

Servings: 1    Cooking Time: 0 Minutes
**Ingredients:**
- ¼ Cup Red Onion, Chopped
- 1 Cup Corn Kernels, Fresh
- 1 Cup Edamame Beans, Shelled & Thawed
- 1 Red Bell Pepper, Chopped
- 2-3 Tablespoons Lime Juice, Fresh
- 5-6 Basil Leaves, Fresh & Sliced
- 5-6 Mint Leaves, Fresh & Sliced
- Sea Salt & Black Pepper to Taste

**Directions:**
Place everything into a Mason jar, and then seal the jar tightly. Shake well before serving. Interesting Facts: Whole corn is a fantastic source of phosphorus, magnesium, and B vitamins. It also promotes healthy digestion and contains heart-healthy antioxidants. It is important to seek out organic corn in order to bypass all of the genetically modified product that is out on the market.
**Nutrition Info:**Calories: 299 Protein: 20 Grams Fat: 9 Grams Carbs: 38 Grams

## Summer Chickpea Salad

Servings: 4    Cooking Time: 15 Minutes
**Ingredients:**
- 1 ½ Cups Cherry Tomatoes, Halved
- 1 Cup English Cucumber, Slices
- 1 Cup Chickpeas, Canned, Unsalted, Drained & Rinsed
- ¼ Cup Red Onion, Slivered
- 2 Tablespoon Olive Oil
- 1 ½ Tablespoons Lemon Juice, Fresh
- 1 ½ Tablespoons Lemon Juice, Fresh
- Sea Salt & Black Pepper to Taste

**Directions:**
Mix everything together, and toss to combine before serving.
**Nutrition Info:**Calories: 145 Protein: 4 Grams Fat: 7.5 Grams Carbs: 16 Grams

## Herbed Risotto

Servings: 4    Cooking Time: 25 Minutes
**Ingredients:**
- cups cauliflower rice
- scallions, chopped
- tablespoons avocado oil
- cups veggie stock
- Juice of 1 lime
- 1 tablespoon parsley, chopped
- 1 tablespoon cilantro, chopped
- 1 tablespoon basil, chopped
- 1 tablespoon oregano, chopped
- 1 teaspoon sweet paprika
- A pinch of salt and black pepper

**Directions:**
Heat up a pan with the oil over medium heat, add the scallions and sauté for 5 minutes. Add the cauliflower rice, the stock and the other ingredients, toss, cook over medium heat for 20 minutes, divide between plates and serve as a side dish.
**Nutrition Info:**Calories 182 fat 4 fiber 2 carbs 8 protein 10

## Roasted Radish With Fresh Herbs

Servings: 4    Cooking Time: 30 Minutes
**Ingredients:**
- 1 tbsp. coconut oil
- 1 bunch radishes
- 2 tbsps. Minced chives
- 1 tbsp. minced rosemary
- 1 tbsp. minced thyme

**Directions:**
Wash the radishes, then remove the tops and stems. Cut them into quarters and reserve. Add the oil to a cast iron pan, then heat to medium. Add the radishes, then season with salt and pepper. Cook on medium heat for 6-8 minutes, until almost tender, then add the herbs and cook through. The radishes can be served warm with meats or chilled with salads.
**Nutrition Info:**Net carbs: 1.8g, Protein: .9g, Fat: 13g, Calories: 133kcal.

## Rib Eyes With Broccoli

Servings: 4    Cooking Time: 15 Minutes
**Ingredients:**
- 4 ounces butter
- ¾ pound Ribeye steak, sliced
- 9 ounces broccoli, chopped
- 1 yellow onion, sliced
- 1 tablespoon coconut aminos
- 1 tablespoon pumpkin seeds
- Salt and pepper to taste

**Directions:**
Slice steak and the onions Chop broccoli, including the stem parts Take a frying pan and place it over medium heat, add butter and let it melt Add meat and season accordingly with salt and pepper Cook until both sides are browned Transfer meat to a platter Add broccoli and onion to the frying pan, add more butter if needed Brown Add coconut aminos and return the meat Stir and season again Serve with a dollop of butter with a sprinkle of pumpkin seeds Enjoy!
**Nutrition Info:**Calories: 875 Fat: 75g Carbohydrates: 8g Protein: 40g

## Salmon, Quinoa, And Avocado Salad

Servings: 4     Cooking Time: 20 Minutes
**Ingredients:**
- ½ cup quinoa
- 1 cup water
- 4 (4-ounce) salmon fillets
- 1-pound asparagus, trimmed
- 1 teaspoon extra-virgin olive oil, plus 2 tablespoons
- ½ teaspoon salt, divided
- ½ teaspoon freshly ground black pepper, divided
- ¼ teaspoon red pepper flakes
- 1 avocado, chopped
- ¼ cup chopped scallions, both white and green parts
- ¼ cup chopped fresh cilantro
- 1 tablespoon minced fresh oregano
- Juice of 1 lime

**Directions:**
In a small pot, combine the quinoa and water, and bring to a boil over medium-high heat. Cover, reduce the heat, and simmer for 15 minutes.     Preheat the oven to 425°F. Line a large baking sheet with parchment paper. Arrange the salmon on one side of the prepared baking sheet. Toss the asparagus with 1 teaspoon of olive oil, and arrange on the other side of the baking sheet. Season the salmon and asparagus with ¼ teaspoon of salt, ¼ teaspoon of pepper, and the red pepper flakes. Roast for 12 minutes until browned and cooked through.     While the fish and asparagus are cooking, in a large mixing bowl, gently toss the cooked quinoa, avocado, scallions, cilantro, and oregano. Add the remaining 2 tablespoons of olive oil and the lime juice, and season with the remaining ¼ teaspoon of salt and ¼ teaspoon of pepper. Break the salmon into pieces, removing the skin and any bones, and chop the asparagus into bite-sized pieces. Fold into the quinoa and serve warm or at room temperature.
**Nutrition Info:**Calories: 397 Total Fat: 22g Protein: 29g Carbohydrates: 23g Sugars: 3g Fiber: 8g Sodium: 292mg

## Orange Scallions And Brussels Sprouts

Servings: 4     Cooking Time: 25 Minutes
**Ingredients:**
- pound Brussels sprouts, trimmed and halved
- 1 cup scallions, chopped
- Zest of 1 lime, grated
- tablespoon olive oil
- ¼ cup orange juice
- tablespoons stevia
- A pinch of salt and black pepper

**Directions:**
Heat up a pan with the oil over medium heat, add the scallions and sauté for 5 minutes.     Add the sprouts and the other ingredients, toss, cook over medium heat for 20 minutes more, divide the mix between plates and serve.
**Nutrition Info:**Calories 193 Fat 4 Fiber 1 Carbs 8 Protein 10

## Carrot Ginger Soup

Servings: 4     Cooking Time: 20 Minutes
**Ingredients:**
- 1 tablespoon olive oil
- 1 medium yellow onion, chopped
- 3 cups fat-free chicken broth
- 1 pound carrots, peeled and chopped
- 1 tablespoon fresh grated ginger
- ¼ cup fat-free sour cream
- Salt and pepper

**Directions:**
Heat the oil in a large saucepan over medium heat. Add the onions and sauté for 5 minutes until softened. Stir in the broth, carrots, and ginger then cover and bring to a boil     Reduce heat and simmer for 20 minutes. Stir in the sour cream then remove from heat.     Blend using an immersion blender until smooth and creamy. Season with salt and pepper to taste then serve hot.
**Nutrition Info:**Calories 125, Total Fat 3.6g, Saturated Fat 0.5g, Total Carbs 17.2g, Net Carbs 13.6g, Protein 6.4g, Sugar 7.8g, Fiber 3.6g, Sodium 385mg

## Shrimp And Black Bean Salad

Servings: 6     Cooking Time: None
**Ingredients:**
- ¼ cup apple cider vinegar
- 3 tablespoons olive oil
- 1 teaspoon ground cumin
- ½ teaspoon chipotle chili powder
- ¼ teaspoon salt
- 1 pound cooked shrimp, peeled and deveined
- 1 (15-ounce) can black beans, rinsed and drained
- 1 cup diced tomatoes
- 1 small green pepper, diced
- ¼ cup sliced green onions
- ¼ cup fresh chopped cilantro

**Directions:**
Whisk together the vinegar, olive oil, cumin, chili powder, and salt in a large bowl.     Chop the shrimp into bite-sized pieces then add to the bowl.     Toss in the beans, tomatoes, bell pepper, green onion, and cilantro until well combined.     Cover and chill until ready to serve.
**Nutrition Info:**Calories 405, Total Fat 9.5g, Saturated Fat 1.7g, Total Carbs 47.8g, Net Carbs 36.2, Protein 33.1, Sugar 2.8g, Fiber 11.6g, Sodium 291mg

## Spinach & Orange Salad

Servings: 6     Cooking Time: 0 Minutes
**Ingredients:**
- ¼ -1/3 Cup Vegan Dressing
- 3 Oranges, Medium, Peeled, Seeded & Sectioned
- ¾ lb. Spinach, Fresh & Torn
- 1 Red Onion, Medium, Sliced & Separated into Rings

**Directions:**
Toss everything together, and serve with dressing. Interesting Facts: Spinach is one of the most superb green veggies out there. Each serving is packed with 3 grams of protein and is a highly encouraged component of the plant-based diet.
**Nutrition Info:**Calories: 99 Protein: 2.5 Grams Fat: 5 Grams Carbs: 13.1 Grams

## Bacon And Blue Cheese Salad

Servings: 2     Cooking Time: 5-7 Minutes
**Ingredients:**
- 2 and ½ ounces fresh spinach
- 1 red onion, sliced
- 3-4 tablespoons blue cheese, crumbled
- 2 ounces almond nibs
- 5 ounces bacon strips

**Directions:**

114

Fry bacon for 2-3 minutes each side, cut the bacon and keep it on the side    Take your salad plate and place spinach leaves on the bottom    Add sliced onion, cheese, bacon    Top with almond nibs    Use your desired Keto-Friendly salad dressing if needed    Toss and enjoy it!

**Nutrition Info:**Calories: 420    Fat: 35g Carbohydrates: 2g    Protein: 24g

## Baked Salmon Cakes

Servings: 4    Cooking Time: 20 Minutes

**Ingredients:**
- 15 ounces canned salmon, drained
- 1 large egg, whisked
- 2 teaspoons Dijon mustard
- 1 small yellow onion, minced
- 1 ½ cups whole-wheat breadcrumbs
- ¼ cup low-fat mayonnaise
- ¼ cup nonfat Greek yogurt, plain
- 1 tablespoon fresh chopped parsley
- 1 tablespoon fresh lemon juice
- 2 green onions, sliced thin

**Directions:**
Preheat the oven to 450°F and line a baking sheet with parchment.    Flake the salmon into a medium bowl then stir in the egg and mustard.    Mix in the onions and breadcrumbs by hand, blending well, then shape into 8 patties.    Grease a large skillet and heat it over medium heat.    Add the patties and fry for 2 minutes on each side until browned.    Transfer the patties to the baking sheet and bake for 15 minutes or until cooked through.    Meanwhile, whisk together the remaining ingredients.    Serve the baked salmon cakes with the creamy herb sauce.

**Nutrition Info:**Calories 240, Total Fat 12.2g, Saturated Fat 1.4g, Total Carbs 9.3g, Net Carbs 7.8g, Protein 25g, Sugar 1.8g, Fiber 1.5g, Sodium 241mg

## Lighter Shrimp Scampi

Servings: 4    Cooking Time: 15 Minutes

**Ingredients:**
- 11/2 pounds large peeled and deveined shrimp
- ¼ teaspoon salt
- 1/8 teaspoon freshly ground black pepper
- 2 tablespoons olive oil
- 1 shallot, chopped
- 2 garlic cloves, minced
- ¼ cup cooking white wine
- Juice of 1/2 lemon (1 tablespoon)

- ½ teaspoon sriracha
- 2 tablespoons unsalted butter, at room temperature
- ¼ cup chopped fresh parsley
- 4 servings (6 cups) zucchini noodles with lemon vinaigrette

**Directions:**
Season the shrimp with the salt and pepper.    In a medium saucepan over medium heat, heat the oil. Add the shallot and garlic, and cook until the shallot softens and the garlic is fragrant, about 3 minutes. Add the shrimp, cover, and cook until opaque, 2 to 3 minutes on each side. Using a slotted spoon, transfer the shrimp to a large plate.    Add the wine, lemon juice, and sriracha to the saucepan, and stir to combine. Bring the mixture to a boil, then reduce the heat and simmer until the liquid is reduced by about half, 3 minutes. Add the butter and stir until melted, about 3 minutes. Return the shrimp to the saucepan and toss to coat. Add the parsley and stir to combine.    Into each of 4 containers, place 11/2 cups of zucchini noodles with lemon vinaigrette, and top with ¾ cup of scampi.

**Nutrition Info:**calories: 364; total fat: 21g; saturated fat: 6g; protein: 37g; total carbs: 10g; fiber: 2g; sugar: 6g; sodium: 557mg

## Onion And Bacon Pork Chops

Servings: 4    Cooking Time: 45 Minutes

**Ingredients:**
- 2 onions, peeled and chopped
- 6 bacon slices, chopped
- ½ cup chicken stock
- Salt and pepper to taste
- 4 pork chops

**Directions:**
Heat up a pan over medium heat and add bacon    Stir and cook until crispy    Transfer to bowl    Return pan to medium heat and add onions, season with salt and pepper    Stir and cook for 15 minutes    Transfer to the same bowl with bacon    Return the pan to heat (medium-high) and add pork chops    Season with salt and pepper and brown for 3 minutes    Flip and lower heat to medium    Cook for 7 minutes more    Add stock and stir cook for 2 minutes    Return the bacon and onions to the pan and stir cook for 1 minute    Serve and enjoy!

**Nutrition Info:**Calories: 325    Fat: 18g Carbohydrates: 6g    Protein: 36g

# Appendix : Recipes Index

Tofu With Brussels Sprouts 79
Tofu With Peas 75
Tomato & Cheese In Lettuce Packets 102
Tomato And Zucchini Sauté 19
Tomato Olive Fish Fillets 63
Tomato Risotto 108
Tortilla Chip With Black Bean Salad 62
Trout Bake 64
Tuna Avocado Salad 111
Tuna Carbonara 61
Tuna Salad 59
Tuna Sweet Corn Casserole 62
Turkey And Spring Onions Mix 51
Turkey With Lentils 51
Turkey-broccoli Brunch Casserole 17
Turkish Tuna With Bulgur And Chickpea Salad 64
Tzatziki Dip With Cauliflower 103

**V**

Vanilla Mixed Berry Smoothie 20
Vegan Cream Soup With Avocado & Zucchini 83
Vegetable And Bean Stew 69

Vegetable And Egg Muffins 33
Vegetable Chicken Soup 86
Vegetable Frittata 22
Vegetable Noodles Stir-fry 15
Vegetable Omelet 22
Vegetables With Irish Beef Roast 37
Vegetarian Split Pea Soup In A Crock Pot 82
Veggie Frittata 21
Veggie Stew 77

**W**

White Spinach Pizza With Cauliflower Crust 107
Whole Roasted Chicken 46
Whole-grain Pancakes 21

**Y**

Yogurt And Kale Smoothie 13
Yogurt Cheesecake 105

**Z**

Zoodle Won-ton Soup 92
Zucchini Risotto 112
Zucchini With Tomatoes 80
Zucchini-basil Soup 85

Made in the USA
Middletown, DE
29 January 2021

32562086R00071